G000126006

Keto diet

And

Keto Chaffle Cookbook

2 Books in 1

The Most Complete Ketogenic Diet Book With Recipes To Lose Weight and Improve Your Health With Delicious Keto Chaffles Recipes

By

Camila Rivera

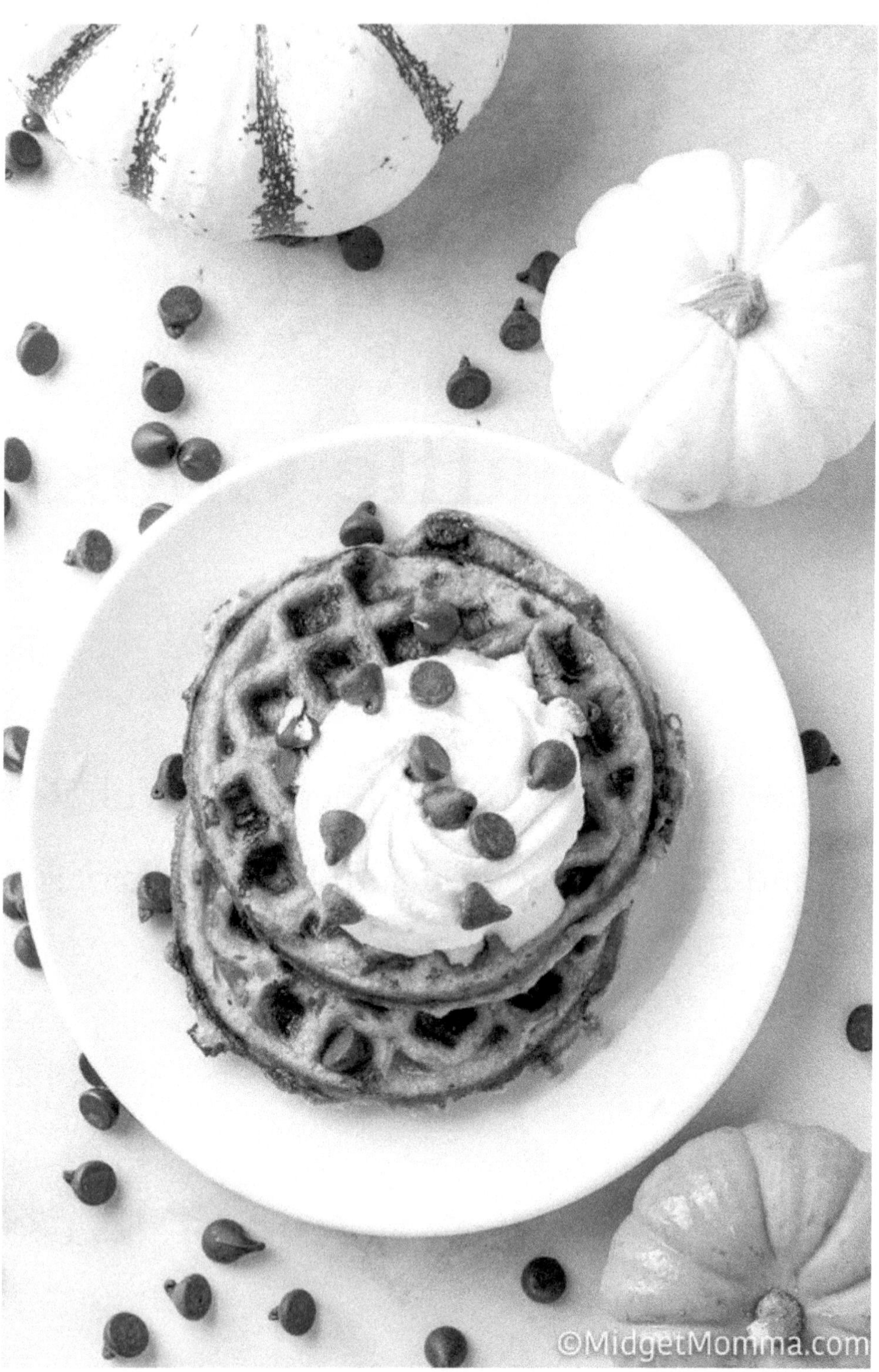
©MidgetMomma.com

© Copyright 2021 - All rights reserved.

This document is geared towards providing exact and reliable information in regards to the topic and issue covered. The publication is sold with the idea that the publisher is not required to render accounting, officially permitted, or otherwise, qualified services. If advice is necessary, legal or professional, a practiced individual in the profession should be ordered.

- From a Declaration of Principles which was accepted and approved equally by a Committee of the American Bar Association and a Committee of Publishers and Associations.

In no way is it legal to reproduce, duplicate, or transmit any part of this document in either electronic means or in printed format. Recording of this publication is strictly prohibited, and any storage of this document is not allowed unless with written permission from the publisher. All rights reserved.

The information provided herein is stated to be truthful and consistent, in that any liability, in terms of inattention or otherwise, by any usage or abuse of any policies, processes, or directions contained within is the solitary and utter responsibility of the recipient reader. Under no circumstances will any legal responsibility or blame be held against the publisher for any reparation, damages, or monetary loss due to the information herein, either directly or indirectly.

Respective authors own all copyrights not held by the publisher.

The information herein is offered for informational purposes solely and is universal as so. The presentation of the information is without contract or any type of guarantee assurance.

The trademarks that are used are without any consent, and the publication of the trademark is without permission or backing by the trademark owner. All trademarks and brands within this book are for clarifying purposes only and are the owned by the owners themselves, not affiliated with this document.

TABLE OF CONTENTS

KETO DIET

KETO CHAFFLE COOKBOOK

Keto diet

An essential guide to begin a keto lifestyle With Quick & Easy Low-Carb Homemade Cooking

By

Camila Rivera

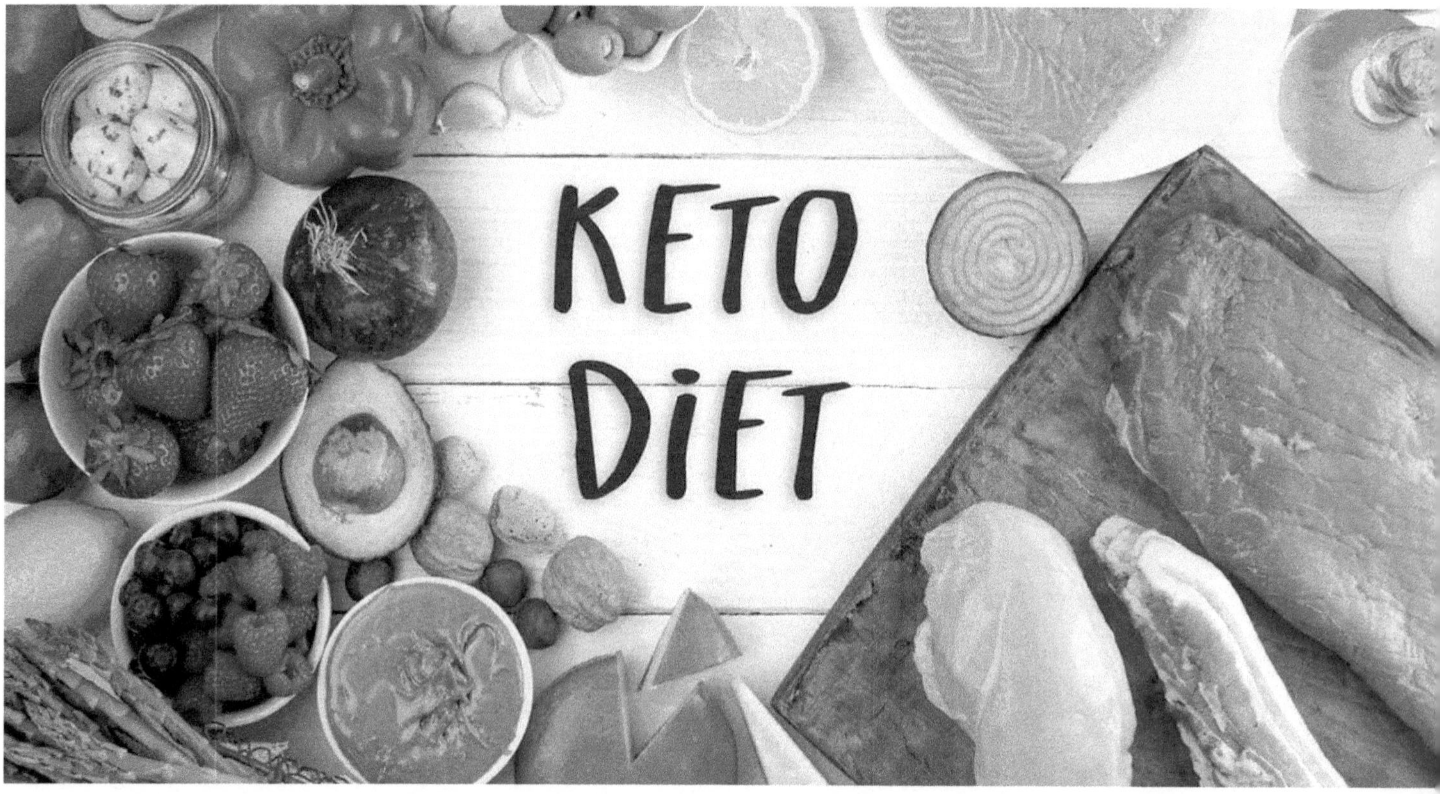
KETO
DiET

Introduction

Ketogenic refers to a low-carbohydrate diet. The aim is to eat more calories from fat and protein while eating fewer calories from carbohydrates. The carbohydrates that are easiest to digest, such as starch, pastries, soda, and white bread, are the first to go. When you consume fewer than 50 g of carbohydrates a day, your body easily runs out of energy. This normally takes three or four days. Then you'll begin to break down fat and protein for energy, potentially resulting in weight loss. Ketosis is the term for this state. It's crucial to remember that the ketogenic diet is a short-term diet designed to help you lose weight rather than change your lifestyle. A ketogenic diet is more often used to reduce weight, although it may also be used to treat medical problems such as epilepsy. It can even benefit those suffering from heart failure, some brain disorders, and even acne, although further study is required. Since the keto diet contains too much fat, adherents must ingest fat at every meal time. In a normal 2K-calorie diet, that would seem like 165 g of fat, 40 g of carbohydrates, and 75 g of protein. The exact ratio, on the other hand, is determined by your basic requirements. Nuts (walnuts, almonds), avocados, seeds, olive oil and tofu are among the healthier unsaturated fats allowed on the keto diet. However, oils (coconut, palm), butter, lard, and peanut butter all contain high amounts of saturated fats. Protein is an essential aspect of the keto diet, although it is also difficult to discern between protein items that are lean and protein products rich in fat(saturated), such as beef, bacon, and pork. What for fruits and vegetables? While fruits are generally rich in carbohydrates, unique fruits may be obtained in limited quantities (generally berries) Leafy greens (like kale, chard, Swiss chard, and spinach), broccoli, cauliflower, asparagus, tomatoes, brussels sprouts, bell peppers, garlic, cucumbers, mushrooms, summer squashes, as well as celery are also rich in carbohydrates. One cup of sliced broccoli includes about six carbohydrates. At the same time, there are several possible keto hazards, such as liver deficiency, liver complications, constipation, kidney disorders, and so on. As a result, we can also keep our Keto diet portions in check.

Understanding The Ketogenic Diet

This chapter delves into the Ketogenic diet in depth. The chapter further discusses which foods to consume on the Keto diet and which foods to stop while on this diet. The Keto diet is often explained in-depth, including how it functions and what health advantages it provides.

The ketogenic diet (or keto diet) is a high-fat, low-carbohydrate diet with various health benefits. Evidently, more than 20 studies suggest that this form of diet will help you lose weight and boost your wellbeing. Diabetes patients, epilepsy patients, patients suffering from Alzheimer's disease, as well as cancer can all benefit from ketogenic diets.

1.1 What is Keto?

The ketogenic diet is a very low carbohydrate, high-fat diet that has a lot in common with the Atkins diet and other low-carb diets. It necessitates a significant reduction of carbohydrate consumption and a replacement with fat. This reduction of carbohydrates puts the body into a metabolic condition known as ketosis. As this occurs, the body's energy production of fat-burning skyrockets. In addition, it converts fat into ketones in the liver, which will supply energy to the brain. Ketogenic diets can result in substantial reductions in insulin as well as blood sugar levels. This, along with the increased ketones, has numerous health benefits.

Ketogenic Diets Come in Many Forms

There are a few variations of the ketogenic diet, including:

The traditional ketogenic diet consists of a diet that is low in carbs, mild in protein, and strong in fats. It usually has a 75 percent fat content, a 5% carbohydrate content, and a 20% protein content.

The cyclic ketogenic diet entails high-carb reefed cycles, such as five ketogenic days accompanied by two days of high carbohydrate use.

A ketogenic diet with particular goals: The diet requires carbs to be inserted in between exercises.

Protein-rich ketogenic diet: This is comparable to a normal keto diet, but it contains extra protein. Usually, the ratio is 60 percent fat, 5% sugars, and 35 percent protein.

However, only normal and protein-rich ketogenic diets have been extensively studied. More complex keto diets, such as targeted or cyclic keto, are mainly utilized by bodybuilders and athletes.

Ketogenic Diet Health Benefits

In fact, the keto diet first gained popularity as a means of treating neurological conditions, such as epilepsy. Following that, research has shown that diet can help with a broad variety of health issues:

Heart disease: The keto diet has been found to decrease risk factors such as body fat, blood sugar, HDL cholesterol and blood pressure.

Alzheimer's disease: The ketogenic diet can ease Alzheimer's symptoms while still delaying the disease's progression.

Epilepsy: Research has demonstrated that a ketogenic diet can significantly reduce seizures in children with epileptic seizures.

Cancer: The diet is actually being used to control a number of diseases and to delay tumor development.

Acne: Lower insulin levels, as well as less sugar or fried food diets, will aid acne recovery.

Parkinson's disease: According to one report, diet can help relieve the effects of Parkinson's disease.

Brain injuries: One study found that the diet would also increase concussions and improve recovery after a brain injury.

Polycystic ovary syndrome: A ketogenic diet may help lower insulin levels and can be helpful in the treatment of polycystic ovary syndrome.

What foods can you consume on a ketogenic diet?

The majority of your meals will revolve around the following foods:

- Salmon, mackerel and tuna are representations of fatty fish.
- Look for pastured eggs, whole eggs, or omega-3 eggs.
- Seek for grass-fed butter plus cream wherever possible.
- Red meat, ham, sausage, turkey, bacon, chicken and steak are all examples of meat.
- Non-processed cheese (goat, cheddar, mozzarella, blue, or cream).
- Flax seeds, walnuts, almonds, pumpkin seeds, chia seeds and other nuts and beans
- Avocado oil, olive oil and coconut oil are the other safe oils.
- Salt, spices and pepper, as well as a variety of herbs, may be used as condiments.
- Avocados: entire avocados or guacamole made freshly.
- Low-carb vegetables including greens, tomatoes, onions, peppers and other related veggies.

Foods to avoid on a ketogenic diet include:

Carbohydrate-rich diets can be avoided as much as possible.

The following is a selection of items that must be eliminated or reduced on a ketogenic diet:

- Sugary drink, ice cream, soda, smoothies, cake, candy and other sugary items
- Wheat, pasta, cereals, rice, and other wheat-based products are examples of starches or grains.
- Sweet potatoes, parsnips, parsnips, potatoes, carrots and other tubers & root vegetables
- Reduced-calorie or low-fat foods are extremely processed and abundant in carbohydrates.
- Fruit: All fruits, with the exception of tiny bits of berries like strawberries.

- Chickpeas, lentils, peas, kidney beans, and other legumes or beans
- Some sauces/condiments: They are also high in unhealthy fat and sugar.
- Unhealthy fats: Limit the intake to mayonnaise, processed vegetable oils, and other processed fats.
- Alcohol: Because of their carb content, certain alcoholic beverages will shake you out of ketosis.
- Dietary ingredients that are sugar-free: Alcohols, which are often rich in sugar, may influence ketone levels in certain situations. These objects seem to have passed through a lot of refining as well.

1.2 What is the Keto diet, and how does it work?

The "ketogenic" keto diet consists of consuming a moderate level of protein, a heavy amount of fat, and relatively little carbohydrates; also, the fruit is forbidden. As for every diet fad, the advantages to adherents include improved vitality, weight reduction, and mental clarity. Is the ketogenic diet, though, what it's cracked up to be?

Dietitians and nutritionists are quiet on the topic. Low-carb diets like keto appear to assist with weight loss in the short term, but they are no more successful than any other self-help or conventional diet. They still don't seem to be enhancing athletic results.

The ketogenic diet was created to treat epilepsy instead of losing weight. In the 1920s, physicians found that holding people on low-carb diets induced their bodies to use fat as the predominant fuel source rather than glucose. When only fat is available for the body to combust or burn, the body converts fats to fatty acids, which are then converted to ketones, which can be used and taken up to power the body's cells.

Currently, feeding the body exclusively ketones prevents epilepsy for unclear causes. However, with the advent of anti-seizure medicines, few patients with epilepsy rely on ketogenic diets anymore, while certain people who may not respond to medications may benefit. Low carb diets like the Atkins diet, which gained popularity in the early

2000s, also spawned keto diets for weight loss. In comparison, all groups of meatier-meal diets restrict carbohydrates. This diet does not have a set structure, although most routines provide for fewer than fifty grams of carbs per day.
A keto diet causes the body to enter a state known as ketosis, in which the body's cells become completely reliant on ketones for nutrition. It's not exactly clear that this leads to weight loss, but ketosis decreases appetite and can affect hunger-controlling hormones, including insulin. As a consequence, proteins and fats can keep humans fuller longer than sugars, resulting in lower net calorie intake.
In one head-to-head comparison, researchers looked at 48 separate diet trials in which subjects were randomly allocated to one of the well-known diets. Low-carb diets like South Beach, Atkins, and Zone, as well as low-fat diets like Ornish diets and portion restriction diets like Weight Watchers and Jenny Craig, were among the options.
Every diet resulted in greater weight loss than almost no diet after six months, according to the results. Low-carb and low-fat dieters lost almost equal amounts of weight as compared to non-dieters, with low-carb dieters losing 19 pounds on average versus low-fat dieters dropping 17.6 pounds (7.99 kilograms). At 12 months, both diet styles displayed symptoms of dropping off, with low-fat and low-carb dieters being 16 pounds (7.27 kg) smaller on average than non-dieters.
There were few differences in weight reduction within the diets of designated people. This is in line with the practice of recommending every diet that an individual practice in order to lose weight.
Another study of well-known diets discovered the Atkins diet, which results in greater weight loss than merely teaching people about portion control. Nevertheless, several of the scientific researched about this low-carb diet featured licensed dietitians assisting respondents in making food decisions, rather than the self-directed approach used by most people. This has been seen in other diet studies, according to the researchers, and the tests' results seem to be more positive in the real world than the weight loss.
Finally, a simple comparison between low-carb versus low-fat dieting revealed that there was a statistically significant difference in the amount of weight lost over a year.

Low-carbohydrate dieters dropped an average of 13 pounds (6 kg), compared to 11.7 pounds for low-fat dieters (5.3 kg).

Ketogenic diets may help us lose weight, but they are no more successful than other diet methods. Since carbohydrate reserves in the body comprise water molecules, the bulk of the weight lost during the early stages of a ketogenic diet is water weight. This gives the scale an exciting amount at first, but weight reduction slows down with time.

What are the keto effects, and how can they help?

The advantages of a keto diet are close to that of other high-fat, low-carb diets, but it tends to be more successful than centrist low-carb diets. Keto is a low-carb, high-fat diet that maximizes health benefits. However, it will slightly raise the likelihood of complications.

Aid in weight loss

Weight reduction can be improved by converting the body into a fat-burning device. Insulin levels - the hormone that retains fat - are falling rapidly, suggesting that fat burning has risen dramatically. This seems to make it much easier to lose bodyweight without going hungry.

More than thirty high-quality observational studies show that low-carb and keto diets are more effective than other diets at losing weight.

Reverse type 2 diabetes by regulating blood sugar

A ketogenic diet has been shown in research to be successful in the treatment of type 2 diabetes, with total disease reversal occurring in certain instances. It makes perfect sense since keto removes the need for therapy, lowers blood sugar levels, and eliminates the potential negative consequences of high insulin levels.

Since a keto diet will reverse type 2 diabetes, it is likely to be helpful in preventing and reversing pre-diabetes. Keep in mind that "reversal" in this context refers to changing the disease, improving glucose tolerance, and reducing the need for care. It may be so drastically altered that after therapy, blood pressure returns to normal with time. In this context, reversal refers to progressing or deteriorating in the reverse direction of the condition. Changes in your lifestyle, on the other side, just succeed if you bring them into effect. If a person returns to the way of life he or she has before diabetes type 2 appeared and advanced, it is possible that success would return with time.

Improve your mental and physical performance:

Some people use ketogenic diets to boost their mental performance. It's also normal for people to feel more energized while they're in ketosis.

They don't need nutritional carbs for the brain on keto. It runs on ketones 24 hours a day, seven days a week, with a small amount of glucose synthesized in the liver. Carbohydrates are not necessary for the diet. As a result, ketosis leads to a steady flow of food (ketones) to the brain, avoiding significant blood sugar spikes. This will also assist with improved focus and attention, as well as clearing brain fog and improving mental awareness.

Epilepsy Treatment

The keto diet has been used to manage epilepsy since the 19th and 20th centuries and has proved to be effective. It has historically been used mainly for adolescents, although in recent years, it has also proved to be useful to adults. Or, used in conjunction with a keto diet, certain people with epilepsy might be able to take less to no anti-epileptic drugs while being seizure-free. This may help to reduce the drug's adverse effects while still improving cognitive capacity.

Breakfast, Lunch and Dinner Recipes

1 Hot Chocolate

(Ready in about 10 minutes | Serving 1 | Difficulty: Easy)

Per serving: Kcal 173, Fat: 17g, Net Carbs: 5g, Protein: 3g

Ingredients

- 2 tbsp cocoa powder, unsweetened, plus extra for garnish
- 1/4 tsp. of vanilla extract
- 1 1/4 cup of water
- 2 1/2 tsp of keto sugar
- 1/4 cup of heavy cream
- Whipped cream

Instructions

Add cocoa and sugar to a frying pan over moderate flame and whisk. Add 2tbsp water and increase the flame. Add rest of water plus cream and whisk frequently. Add vanilla and stir. Pour mixture in mug and top with whipped cream. Sprinkle cocoa powder and enjoy.

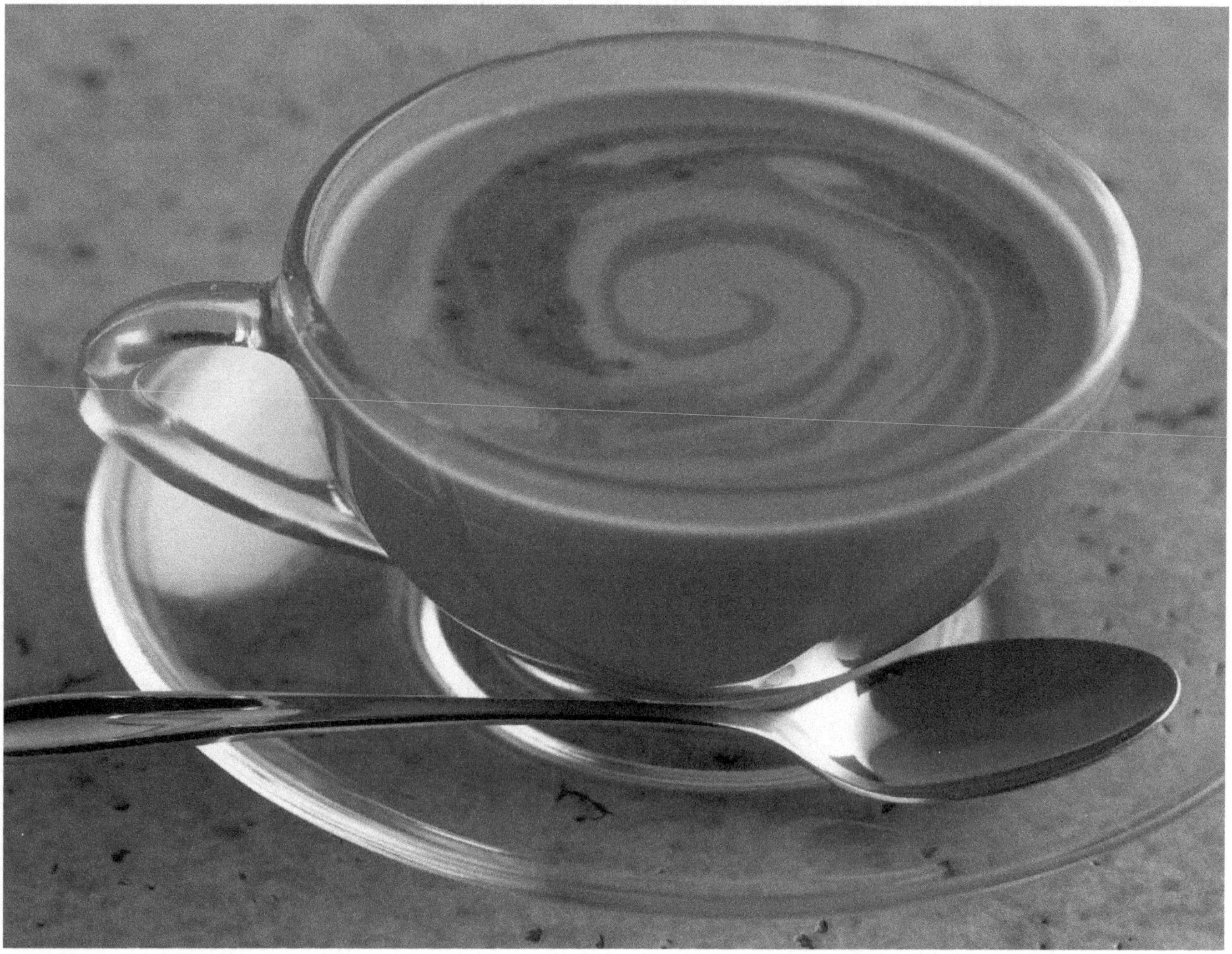

2 Classic bacon with eggs

(Ready in about 10 minutes | Serving 4 | Difficulty: Easy)

Per serving: Kcal 425, Fat: 31g, Net Carbs: 2g, Protein: 33g

Ingredients

- 8 eggs
- cherry tomatoes
- 9 oz. bacon, sliced
- fresh thyme

Instructions

Add bacon to the pan and fry over moderate flame. Add to the plate once it turns crispy and place aside. Fry eggs in the fat left in the pan. Cook to your preference and add tomatoes and cook as well. Add pepper and salt and eat with bacon.

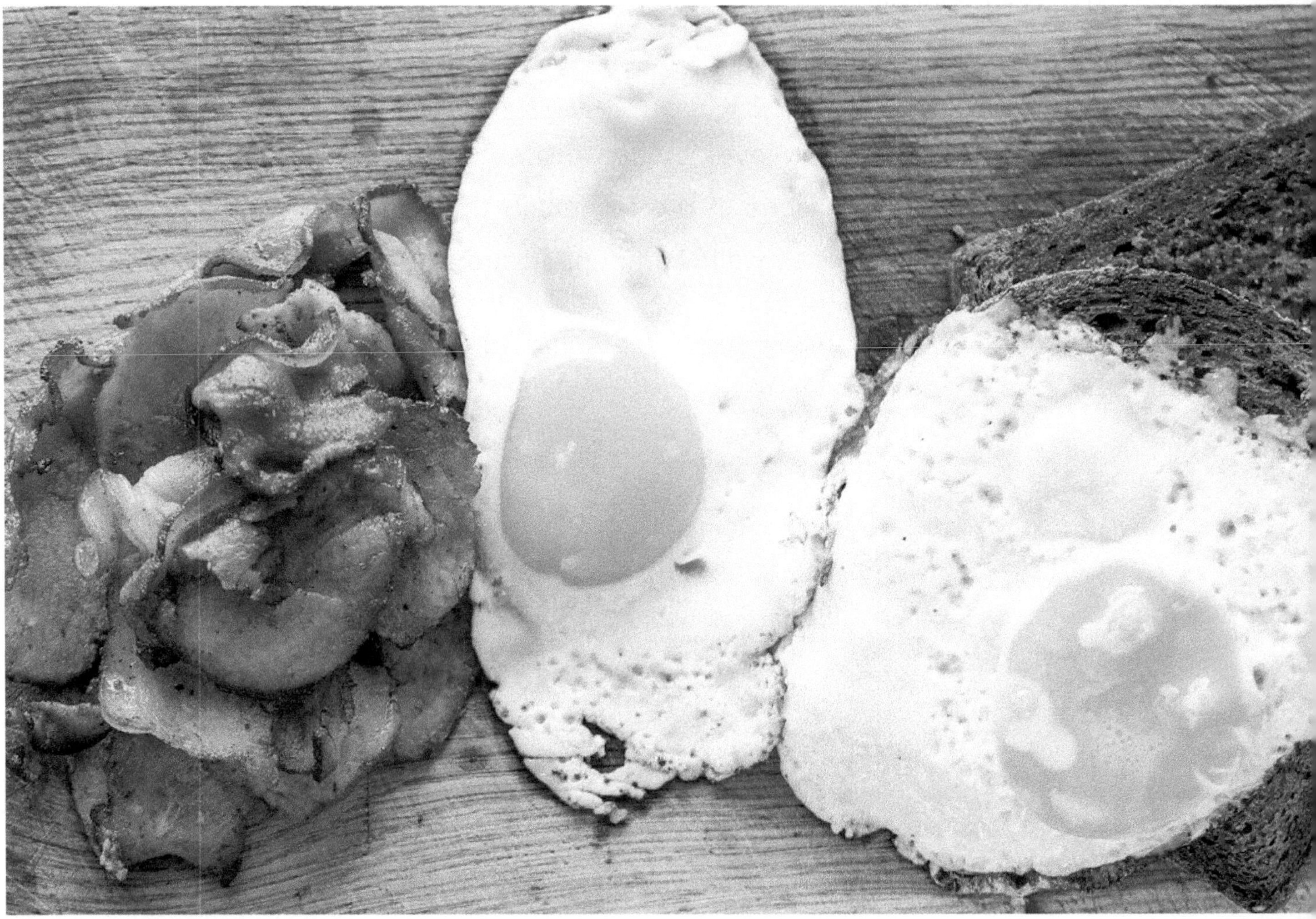

3 keto breakfast

(Ready in about 10 minutes | Serving 1 | Difficulty: Easy)

Per serving: Kcal 424, Fat: 41g, Net Carbs: 1g, Protein: 13g

Ingredients

- 1 cup of baby spinach
- 2 eggs
- 2 tbsp of mayonnaise
- 1 tbsp of butter
- black pepper and salt

Instructions

Warm butter in a pan over moderate flame and add cracked eggs. Cook eggs according to your preference and add pepper and salt over them. Serve with a dollop of mayonnaise plus baby spinach. Have a cup of black coffee along.

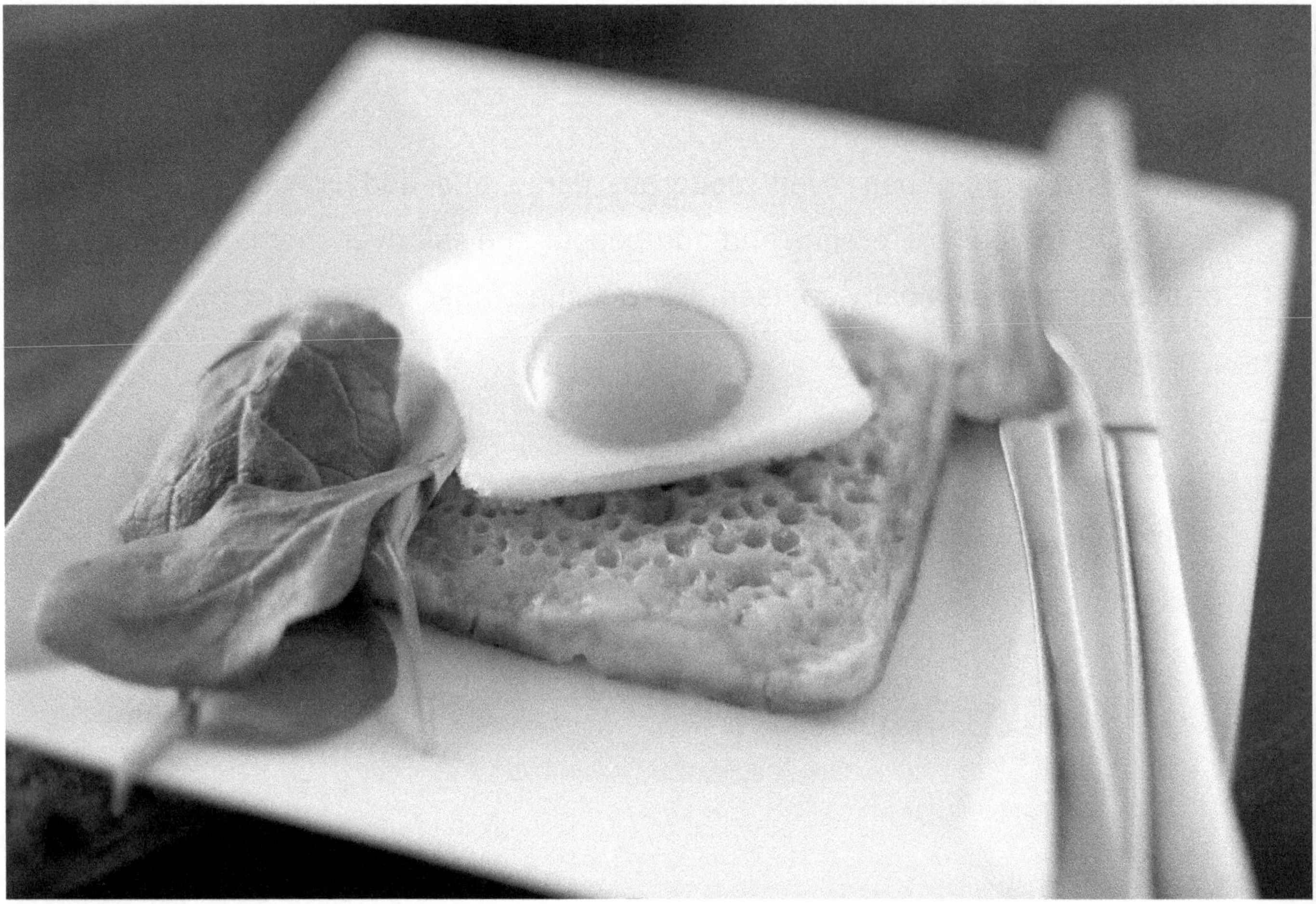

4 Spinach and scrambled eggs

(Ready in about 8 minutes | Serving 1 | Difficulty: Easy)

Per serving: Kcal 368, Fat: 32g, Net Carbs: 2g, Protein: 18g

Ingredients

- 1 tbsp of butter
- black pepper and salt
- 2 eggs
- 2 tbsp of whipping cream
- 1 cup of baby spinach
- 1 oz. salmon smoked

Instructions

Warm butter in a pan over moderate flame and fry baby spinach until it turns soft. Add cream and cook until it bubbles and turns creamy. Breaks eggs into the pan and mix to incorporate all the ingredients. Season using pepper and salt. Continue stirring and cook according to your preference. Add eggs to the pan and serve with smoked salmon.

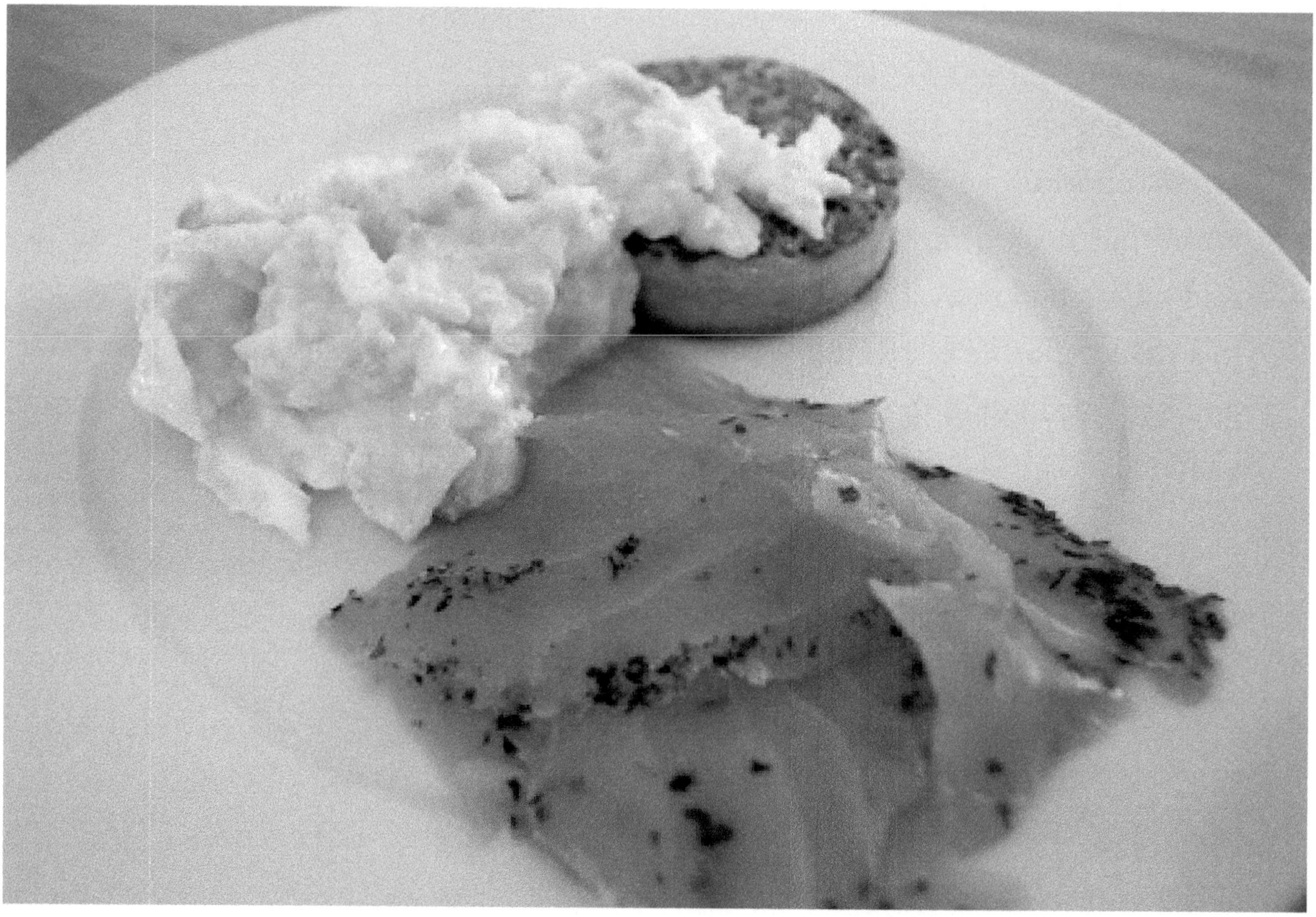

5 Oven pancake

(Ready in about 40 minutes | Serving 4 | Difficulty: Moderate)

Per serving: Kcal 553, Fat: 49g, Net Carbs: 5g, Protein: 22g

Ingredients

- 31/2 oz. pork bacon
- 2 tbsp of butter 4 eggs
- 1 tsp of baking powder
- 2 oz. of yellow onion
- 1 cup of whipping cream
- 1/2 cup of almond flour
- 1/2 cup cottage cheese
- 1 tbsp of husk powder
- 1 tsp of salt

Instructions

Preheat the oven to 350 degrees F. Dice onion and bacon. Warm butter in a pan and cook onion and bacon in the pan until the bacon gets crispy and onion is translucent. Add the rest of the ingredients to a bowl and mix. Pour mixture in a pan and top with onions and bacon. Bake for around 25 minutes and enjoy.

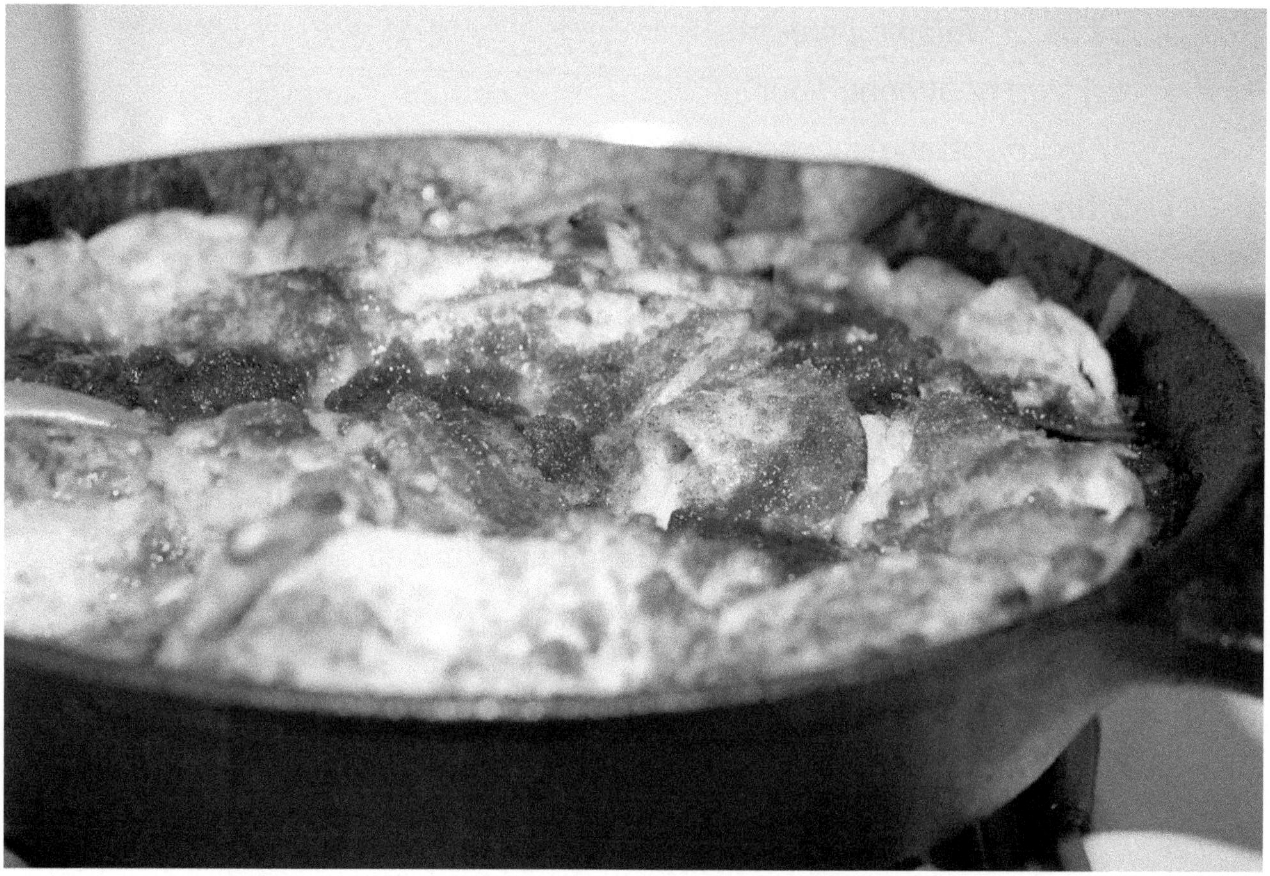

6 Pulled Pork

(Ready in about 20 minutes | Serving 1 | Difficulty: Easy)

Per serving: Kcal 153, Fat: 10, Net Carbs: 8g, Protein: 6g

Ingredients

- 2 tbsp of olive oil
- 1/4 tsp of salt
- 2 eggs
- 1 (115g) diced turnip 1/2 tsp paprika
- 1/4 tsp of garlic powder
- 3 halved(50g) Brussels sprouts
- 1/4 tsp of black pepper
- 1 cup of spinach chopped
- 3 ounces of pulled pork
- 2 tbsp diced red onion
- 1 tbsp of parsley chopped

Instructions

Warm oil in a pan over moderate flame. Add spices and turnip and cook for around 5 minutes.

Add the rest of the veggies and cook for around 3 minutes. Add pork and cook for 2 more minutes. Break eggs and cook for around 5 minutes, covered. Season using pepper and salt and top with parsley.

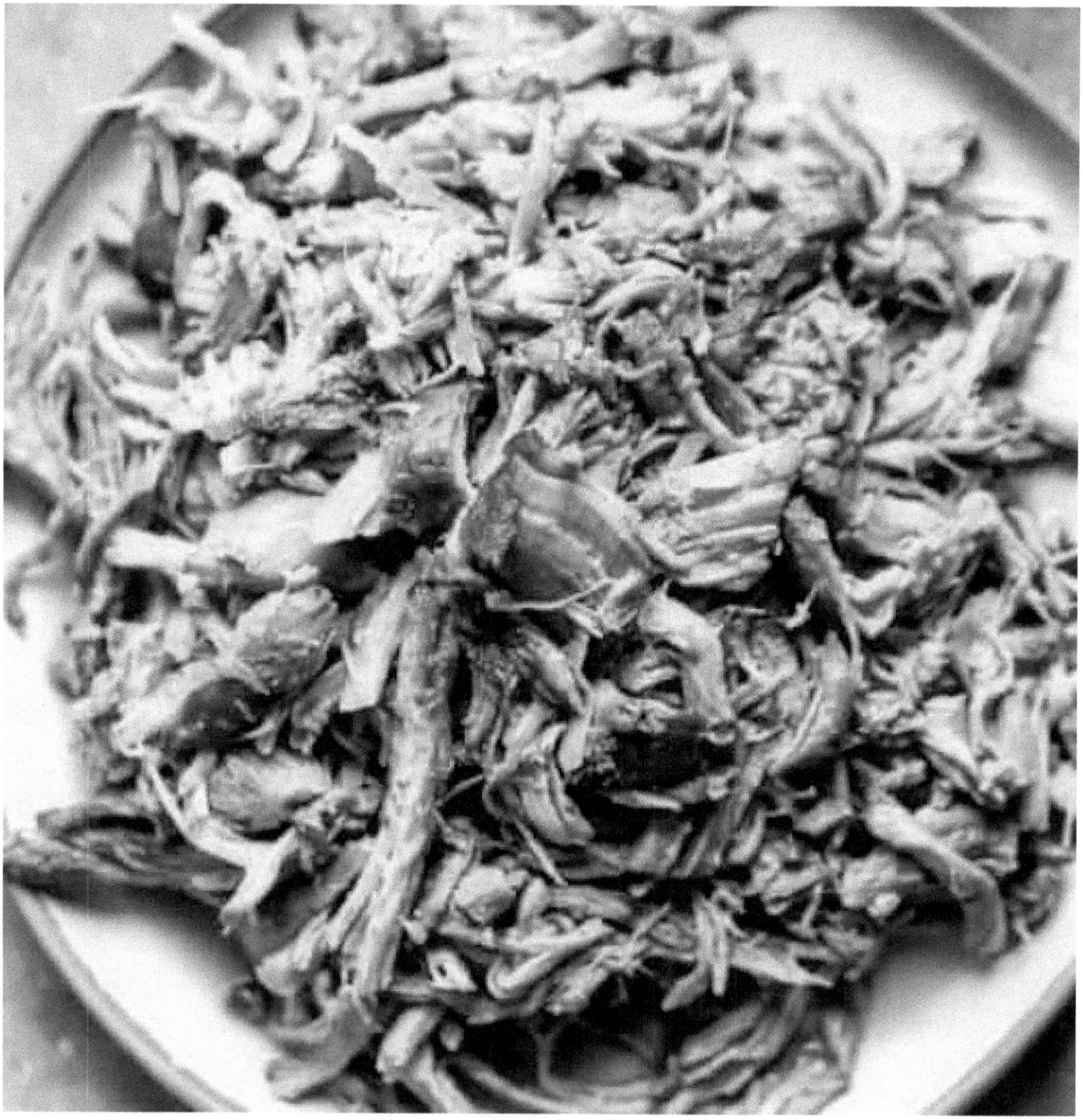

7 Bacon Egg Cups

(Ready in about 30 minutes | Serving 12 | Difficulty: Easy)

Per serving: Kcal 115, Fat: 8g, Net Carbs: 0g, Protein: 9g

Ingredients

- Bacon strips 12
- pepper, to taste
- 12 Big eggs

Instructions

Preheat the oven to 400 degrees F. Spray a muffin tin using cooking spray and place aside. Use one bacon piece for every muffin and form a basket for the egg. Add bacon inside in a way that it covers the sides, and use scissors to remove the extra bacon. Add this to the bottom of the basket and repeat with the rest of the bacon pieces. Bake for around 7 minutes and break an egg in each basket. Bake for another 15 minutes. Season using pepper and enjoy.

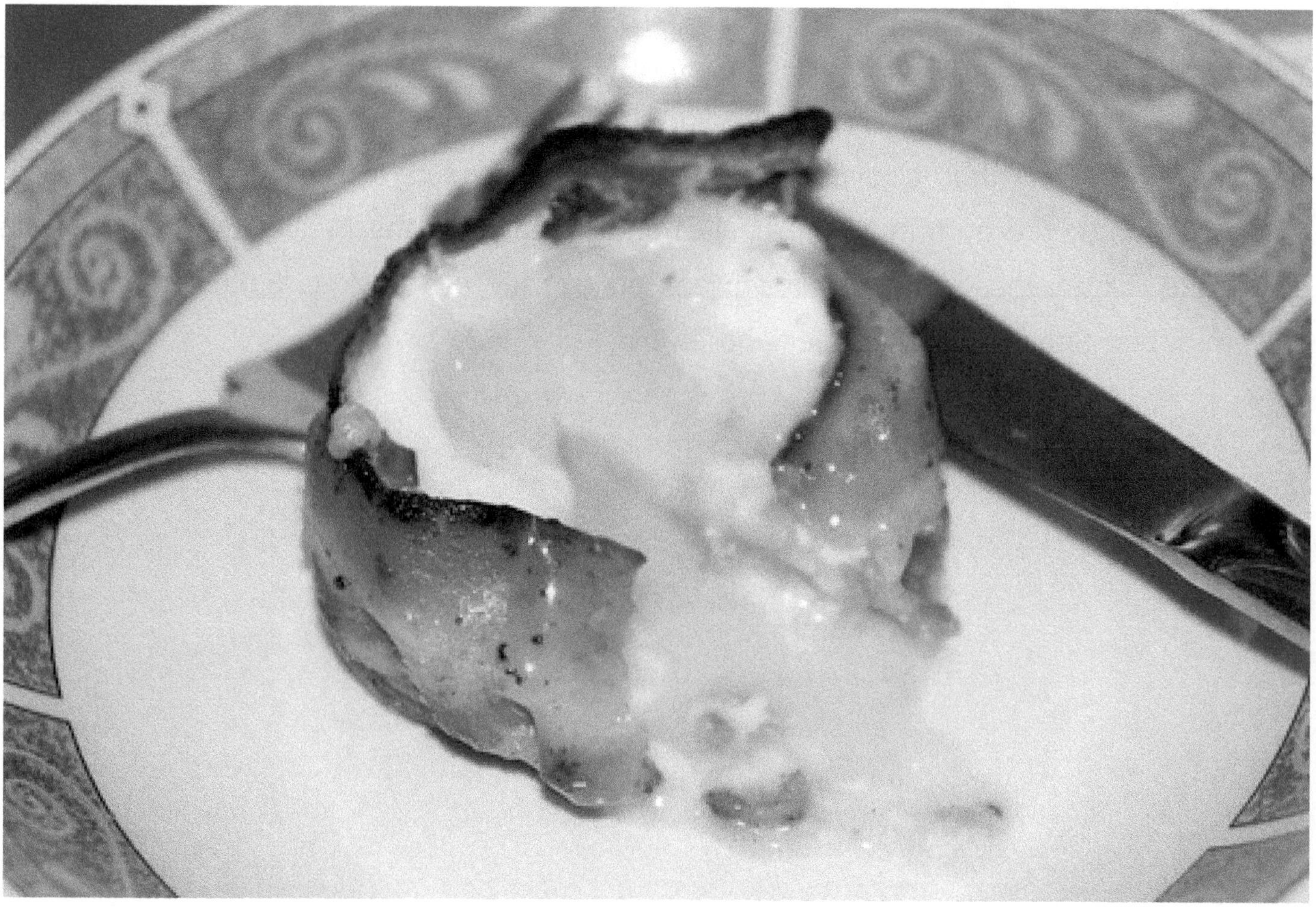

8 Granola Clusters

(Ready in about 45 minutes | Serving 8 | Difficulty: Moderate)

Per serving: Kcal 327, Fat: 31.5, Net Carbs: 6g, Protein: 5.5

Ingredients

- 1 cup of pecan halves
- 1/2 cup of almonds
- 1/4 cup of powdered Sweetener
- 1 cup of flaked coconut
- 1/2 cup of pumpkin seeds
- 1/2 cup of butter
- 1/2 tsp of salt
- 1/4 cup of Swerve Brown
- 1/2 tsp of vanilla extract

Instructions

Preheat the oven to 300 degrees F. Use parchment paper to line a baking dish. Combine everything except sweeteners and butter in a blender and blend. Add sweeteners and butter in a pan placed on low flame. Whish until sweeteners are dissolved, and butter melts. Add nut mixture and mix. Pour mixture in a prepared pan in a single layer. Top with parchment paper and bake for around 30 minutes.

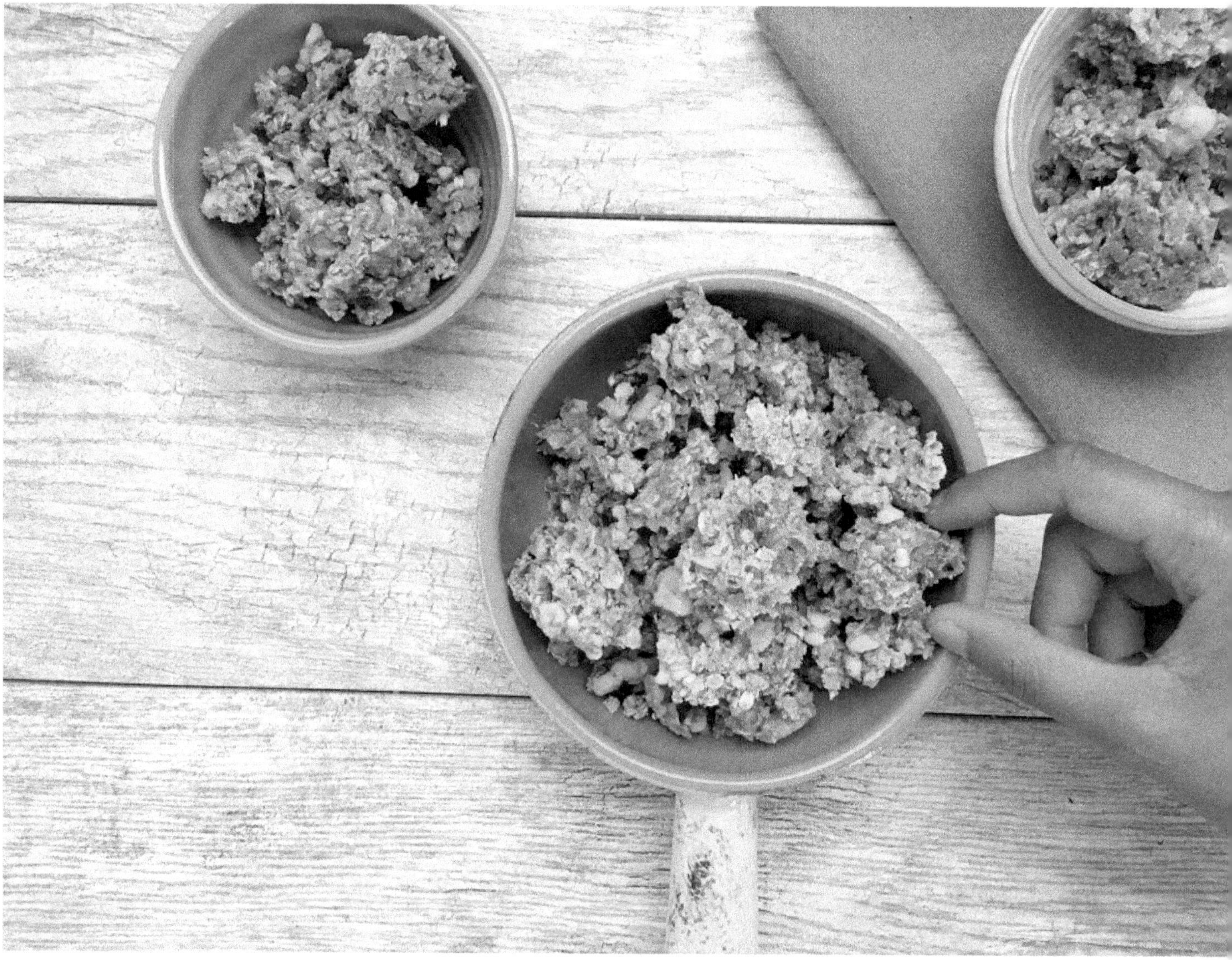

9 Crustless Quiche

(Ready in about 35 minutes | Serving 6 | Difficulty: Moderate)

Per serving: Kcal 216, Fat: 17g, Net Carbs: 4g, Protein: 11g

Ingredients

- 1/2 cup of bacon chopped
- 1/4 tsp of black pepper ground
- 1/2 cup of chopped cherry tomatoes
- 1/2 cup of broccoli chopped
- 1/2 tsp of salt
- 1/2 cup of milk
- 2/3 cup mozzarella cheese shredded
- 1/2 cup of half and half
- 5 eggs

Instructions

Preheat the oven to 325 degrees F. Use cooking spray to spray a baking dish and spread tomatoes, broccoli, plus bacon evenly on the dish. Combine the rest of the ingredients in a bowl and pour over veggies. Sprinkle cheese on top and bake for around 25 minutes.

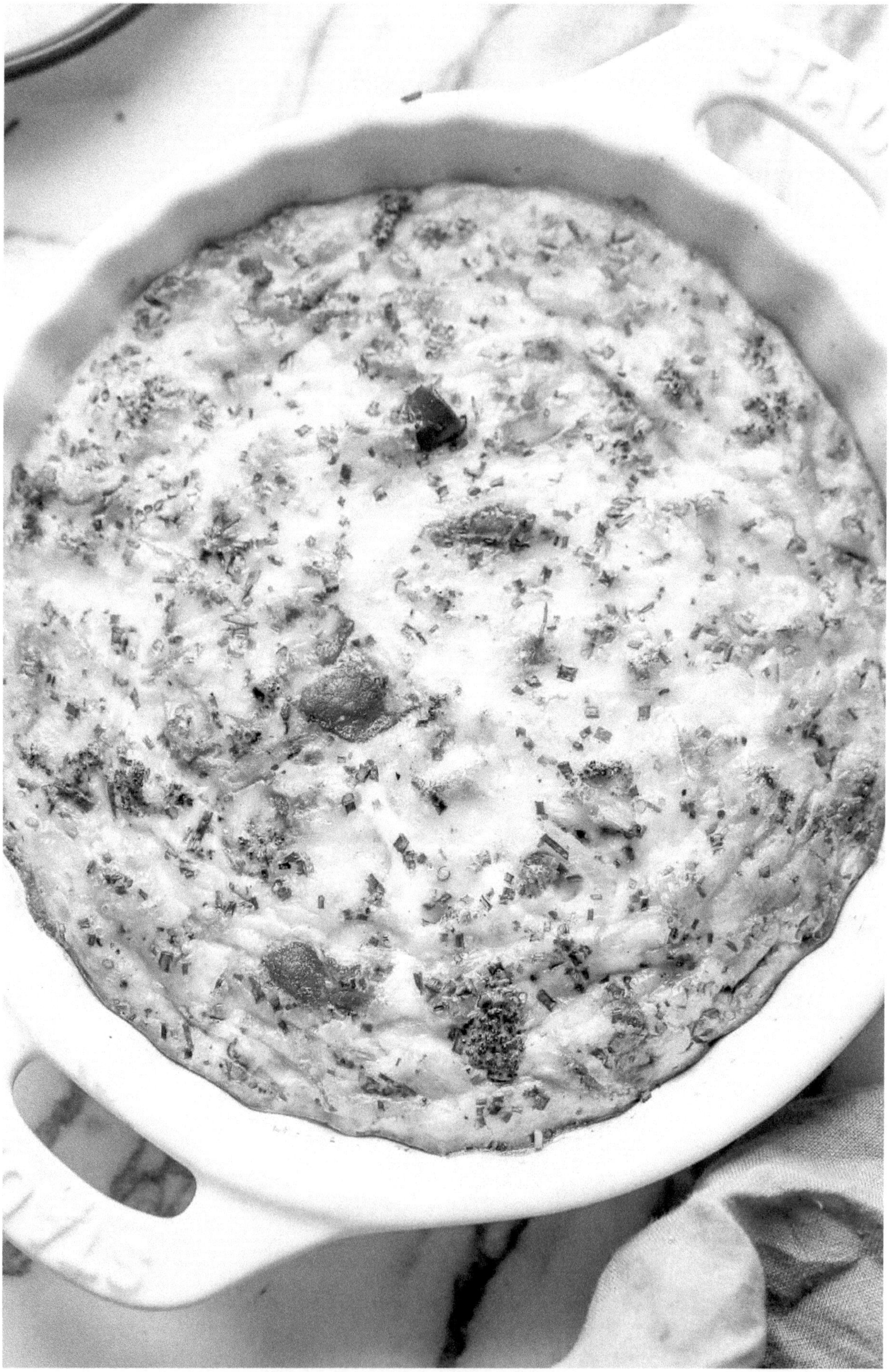

10 Fluffy Eggs

(Ready in about 10 minutes | Serving 4 | Difficulty: Easy)

Per serving: Kcal 281, Fat: 20.2g, Net Carbs: 5.2g, Protein: 19.7g

For Scrambled eggs

- 1 handful of chives
- Black pepper ground
- 4 ounces of goat cheese
- 8 eggs
- 1/2 tsp of kosher salt
- 2 tbsp of butter

Instructions

Dice the chives. Whisk eggs in a bowl and add goat cheese. Add pepper and salt and stir. Warm butter in a pan over moderate flame. Add eggs mixture, and once eggs start to harden, make folds with a spatula by slowly scraping egg sections. Garnish with chives and enjoy.

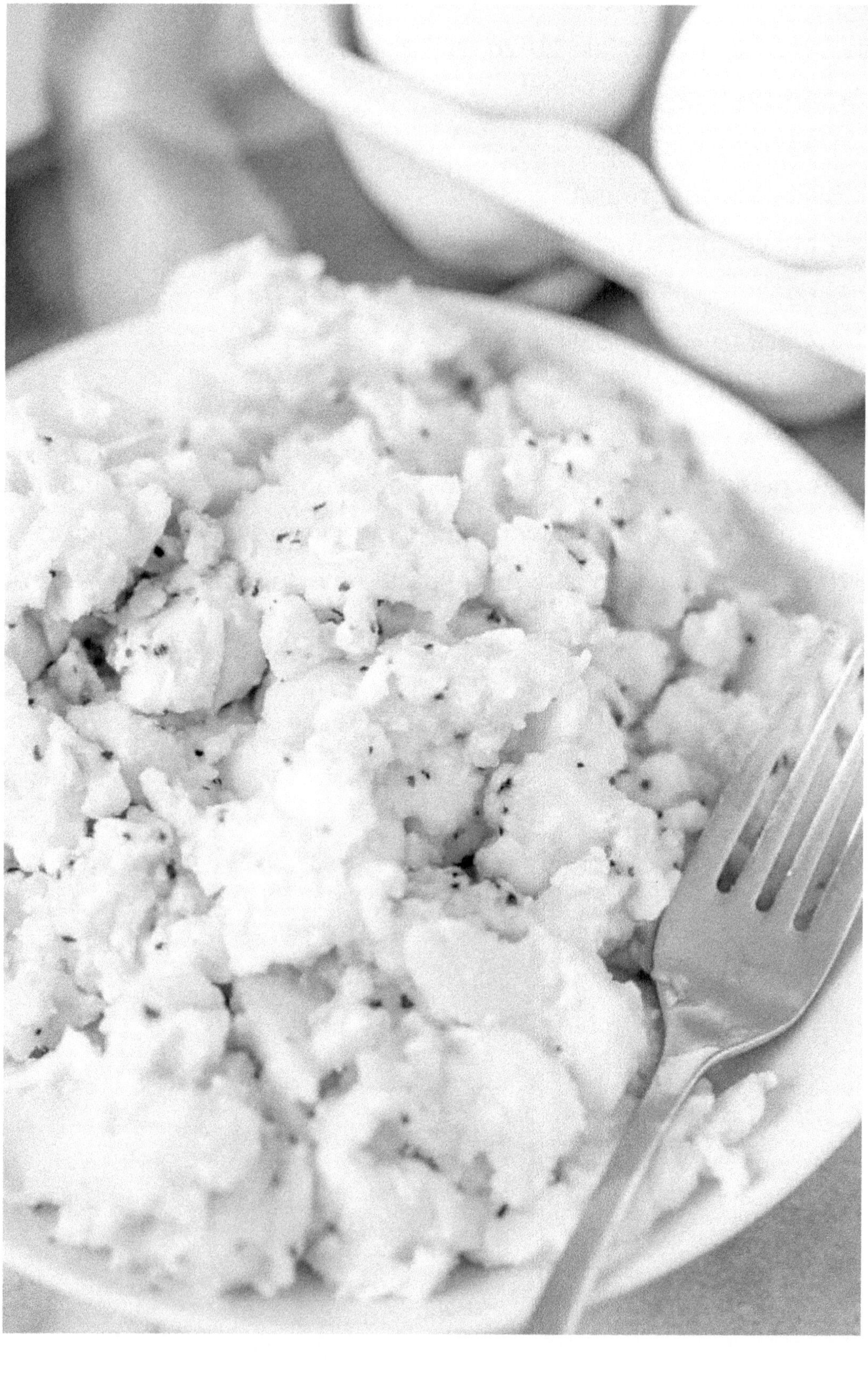

11 Keto Pancakes

(Ready in about 10 minutes | Serving 4 | Difficulty: Easy)

Per serving: Kcal 395, Fat: 34, Net Carbs: 12g, Protein: 14g

Ingredients

- 1 cup of almond flour
- 1/3 cup unsweetened almond milk
- 2-3 tbsp of sweetener of choice
- 1/4 tsp of salt
- 1/4 cup of coconut flour
- 5 large eggs
- 1 tsp of baking powder gluten-free
- 1 1/2 tsp of vanilla extract
- 1/4 cup of coconut oil
- Berries

Instructions

Add all the ingredients to a bowl and mix. Preheat the griddle to approximately 300 degrees F. Pour a quarter of the mixture onto the griddle and heat for around2 minutes. Flip to cook the other side for 2 minutes as well. Repeat with the remaining mixture and enjoy.

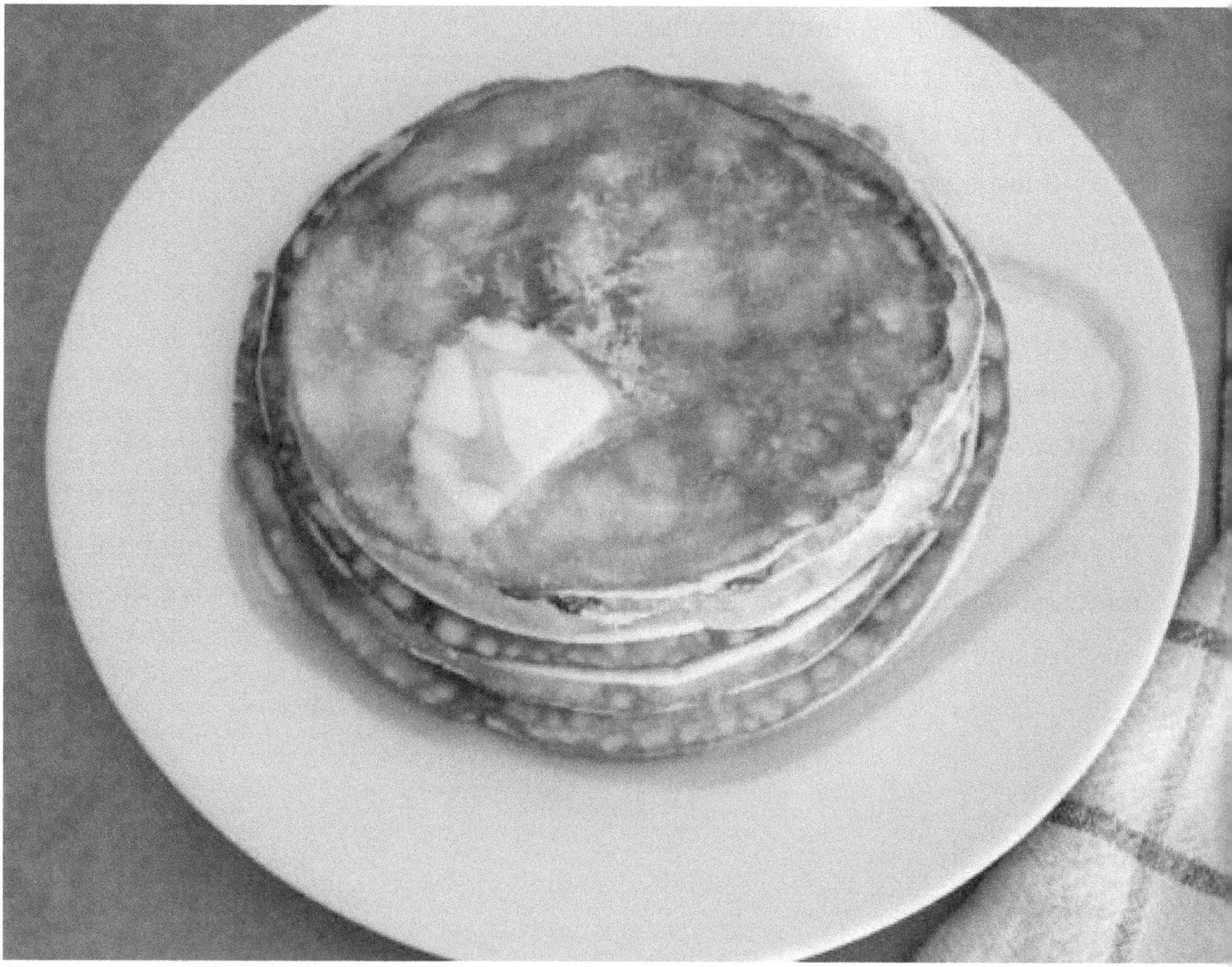

12 Frittata Muffins

(Ready in about 30 minutes | Serving 12 | Difficulty: Easy)

Per serving: Kcal 164, Fat: 14g, Net Carbs: 4g, Protein: 7g

Ingredients

- 4 tbsp of avocado oil
- 3 minced garlic cloves
- 1/2 pound thawed frozen spinach squeezed dry
- 1/2 medium diced onion
- 1/2 pound sliced cremini mushrooms
- 5 ounces of Prosciutto di Parma
- Kosher salt
- 2 tbsp of coconut flour
- 8 Big eggs
- Ground pepper
- 1/4 cup of coconut milk
- 1 cup halved cherry tomatoes

Instructions

Preheat the oven to 375 degrees F. Warm 2 tbsp of avocado oil in a frying pan over moderate flame. Sauté onions until translucent. Add mushrooms and garlic and cook until the moisture from mushrooms evaporates. Season filling using pepper and salt. Transfer to a plate. Beat eggs with the rest of the ingredients in a separate bowl to prepare the batter. Add spinach and mushrooms and mix. Brush muffin tin with remaining avocado oil and use prosciutto to line all cups. Pour frittata batter in every cup and top with diced tomatoes. Bake for around 20 minutes and turn at half point.

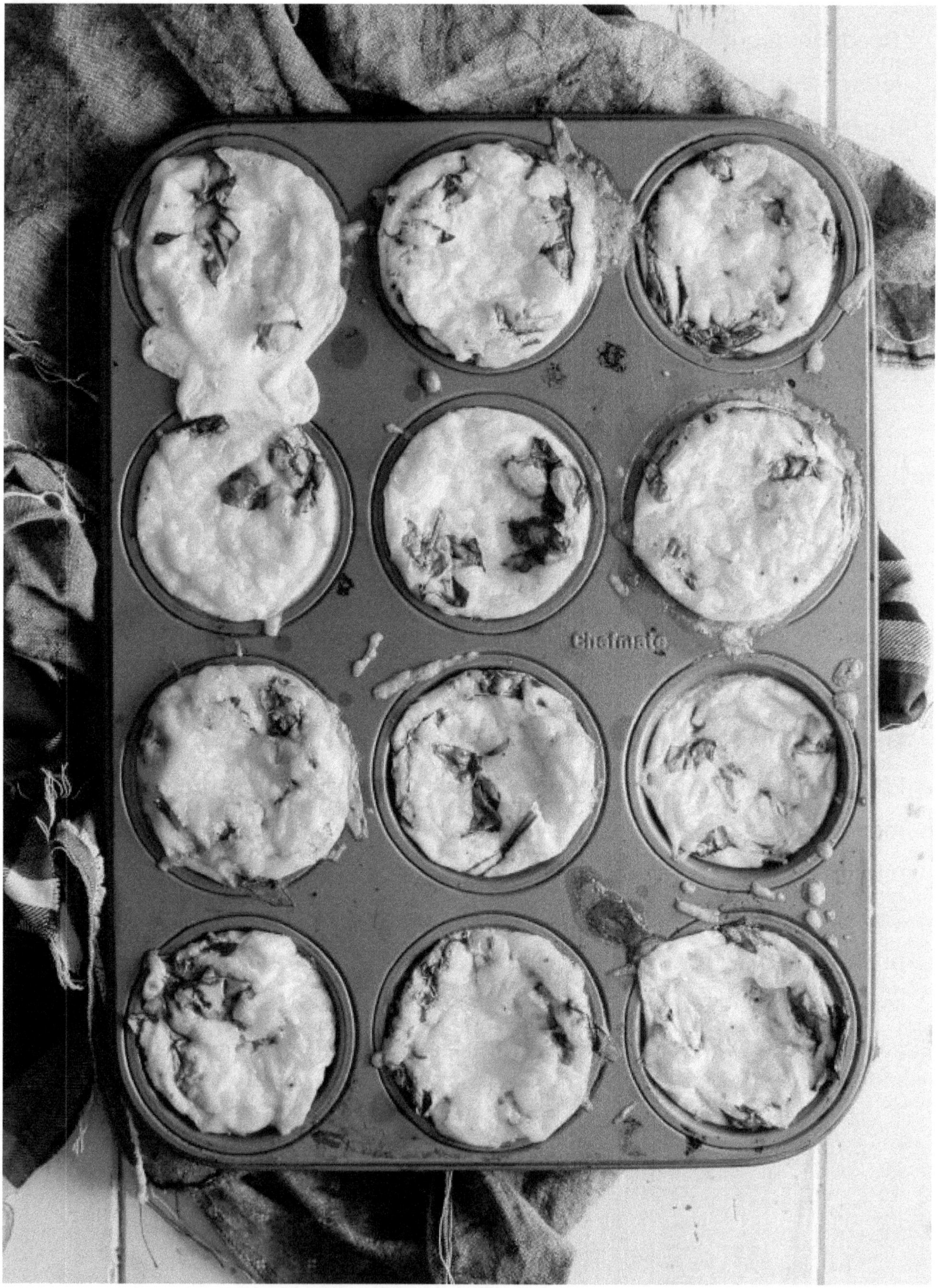

13 Bacon Omelet

(Ready in about 32 minutes | Serving 4 | Difficulty: Easy)

Per serving: Kcal 311, Fat: 20g, Net Carbs: 3g, Protein: 17g

Ingredients

- 8 eggs
- 4 cooked bacon slices chopped
- 1 sliced leek
- 2 tbsp of ghee
- Micro greens
- Black pepper ground and sea salt
- Fresh minced chives

Instructions

Neat eggs in a bowl and season using pepper and salt. Melt ghee in a pan over moderate flame. Cook leek for around 5 minutes in the pan and add cooked bacon plus egg mixture in the pan. Cook until it starts to settle and flip to cook the other side for around 3 minutes. Top with chives and micro greens.

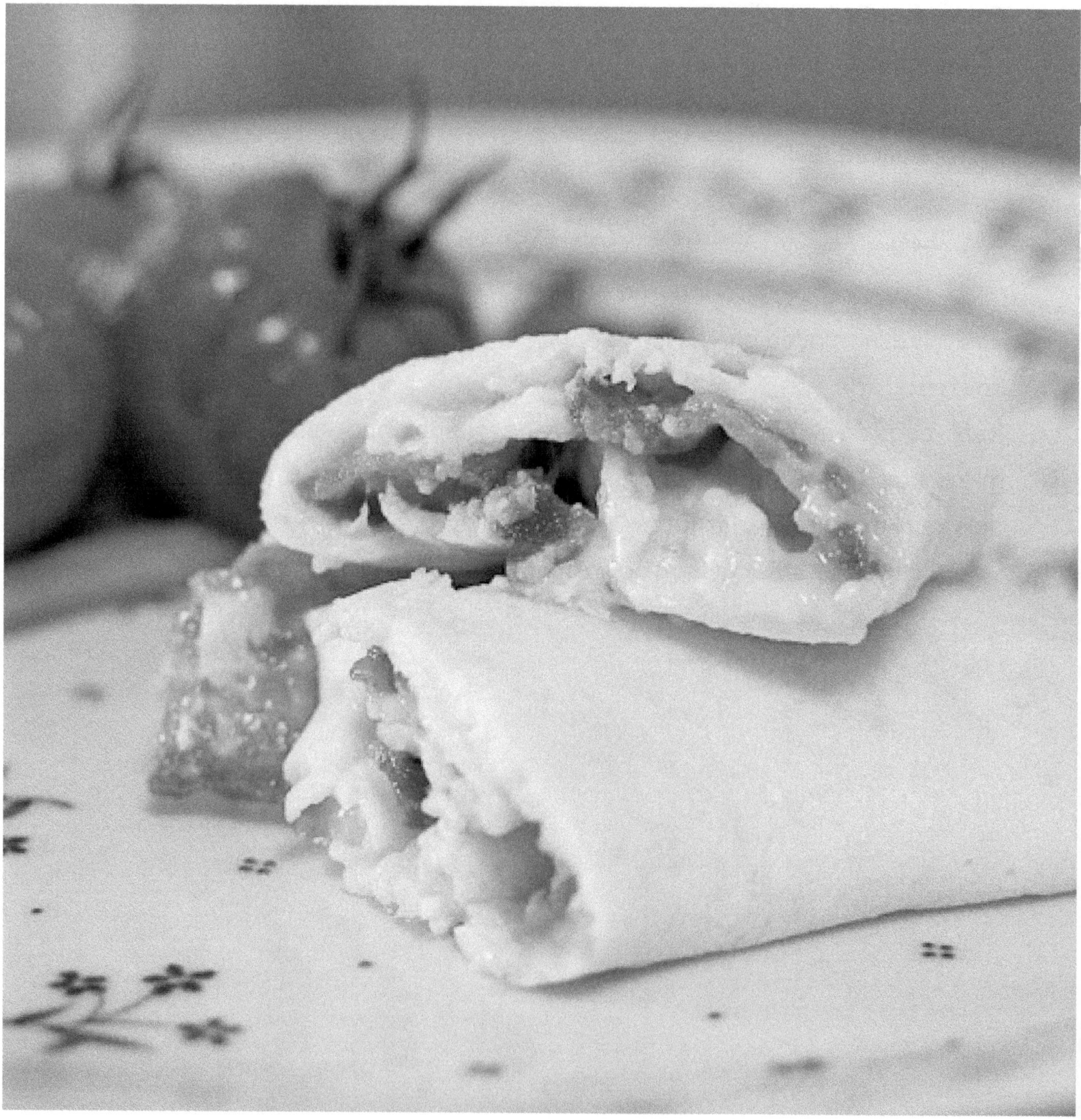

14 Brie Frittata

(Ready in about 25minutes | Serving 6 | Difficulty: Easy)

Per serving: Kcal 338, Fat: 27g, Net Carbs: 1.8g, Protein: 18g

Ingredients

- 8 slices chopped bacon
- 1/2 cup of whipping cream
- 8 Big eggs
- 2 minced cloves garlic
- 1/2 tsp of pepper
- 1/2 tsp of salt
- 4 ounces sliced brie

Instructions

Cook bacon in a pan until it turns crispy. Drain on a plate lined with a paper towel. Whisk eggs with the rest of the ingredients plus bacon(two-thirds). Pour mixture in a pan containing bacon grease and cook until egg at edges set up and is somewhat loose in the center. Layer the diced brie on eggs and sprinkle the rest of the bacon. Preheat the broiler to high temperature and position the oven rack in the oven at the second-highest point. Broil for around 5 minutes.

15 Fried Rice

(Ready in about 30 minutes | Serving 4 | Difficulty: Easy)

Per serving: Kcal 108, Fat: 7g, Net Carbs: 21g, Protein: 13g

Ingredients

- 1 diced into florets cauliflower head
- 1 sliced bunch of scallions
- 2 tbsp of coconut oil
- 3 minced garlic cloves
- 2 peeled carrots, diced
- 1 tbsp fresh ginger minced
- 2 diced celery stalks
- 1 cup of frozen peas
- 1 diced bell pepper
- 2 tbsp of rice vinegar
- 2 tsp of Sriracha
- 3 tbsp of soy sauce

Garnishes

- 1 tbsp coconut oil
- Black pepper ground and sea salt
- 4 tbsp scallions sliced
- 4 eggs
- 4 tbsp fresh cilantro chopped
- 4 tsp of sesame seeds

Instructions

Pulse cauliflower in food processor's bowl for around 3 minutes and place aside. Warm oil in a pan and add ginger, scallions and garlic and cook for around 1 minute. Add celery, bell pepper and carrots and cook for around 11 minutes. Add cauliflower rice and cook for 5 additional minutes. Add frozen peas and mix. Add sriracha, rice vinegar and soy sauce and mix. Place aside. Warm oil in a pan and break eggs in it. Cook for around 4 minutes and season using pepper and salt. Top rice with egg and garnish using 1 tbsp cilantro, tsp sesame seeds and 1 tbsp scallions in four plates.

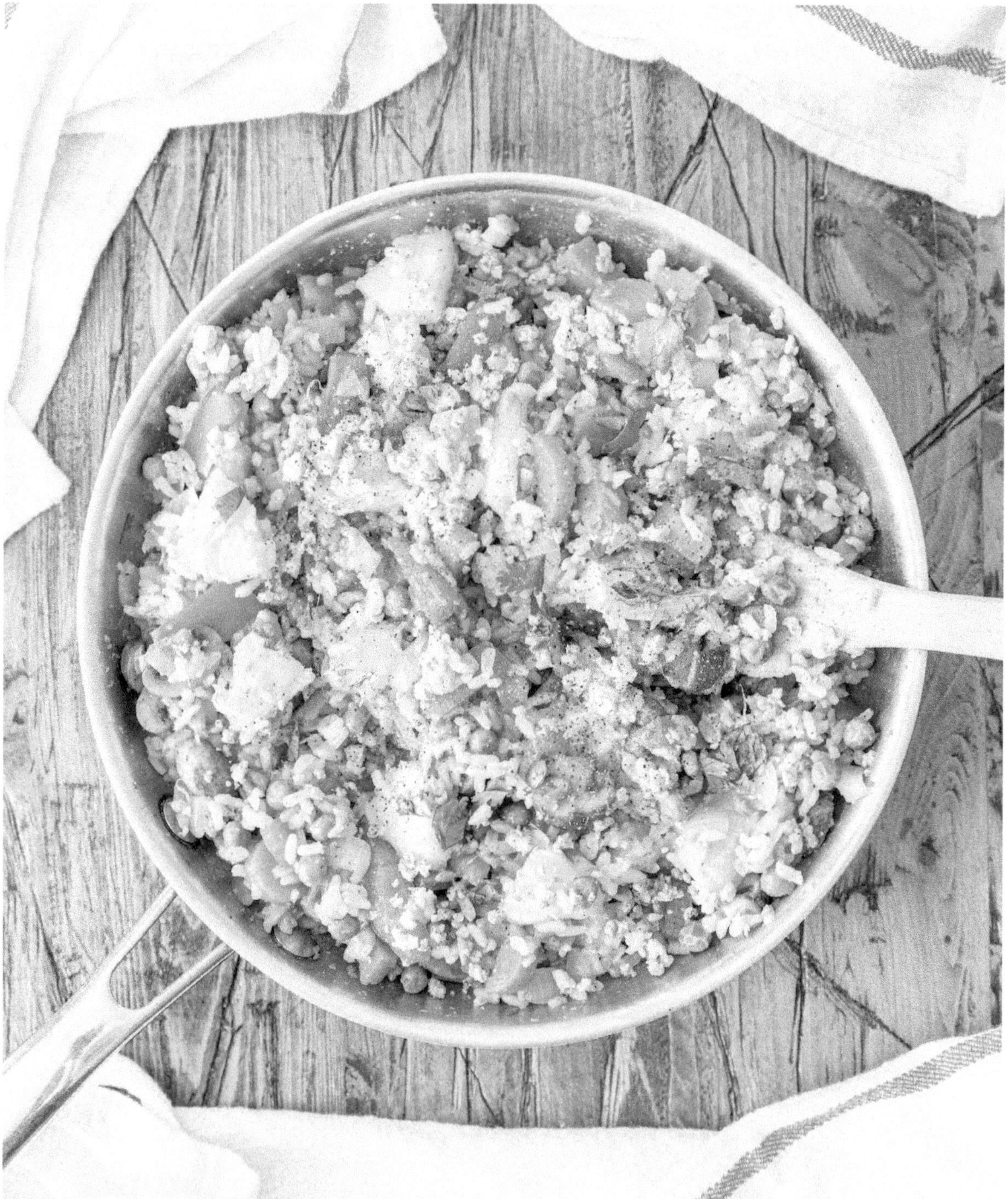

16 Thai Soup

(Ready in about 22 minutes | Serving 6 | Difficulty: Easy)

Per serving: Kcal 323, Fat: 27g, Net Carbs: 7g, Protein: 15g

Ingredients

Main Soup

- 4 Boneless Chicken Thighs skin removed
- 2 tsp of Thai curry paste
- 4 cloves Garlic, crushed
- 14.5 oz of Coconut Milk
- 2 tsp of Fish Sauce
- 1 tsp of Agave nectar
- 3 tsp of Soy Sauce
- 2 Chopped Green Scallions
- 2 inches chopped Minced Ginger

Veggies

- 1/2 cup of sliced cherry tomatoes
- 3 chopped green scallions
- 1/4 cup of chopped cilantro
- 1 lime, juiced

Instructions

Add soup ingredients in an instant pot and close. Cook by pressing the soup button for around 12 minutes under pressure. Release pressure using quick technique and take out chicken shred and add back to the soup. Add vegetables to broth and sear.

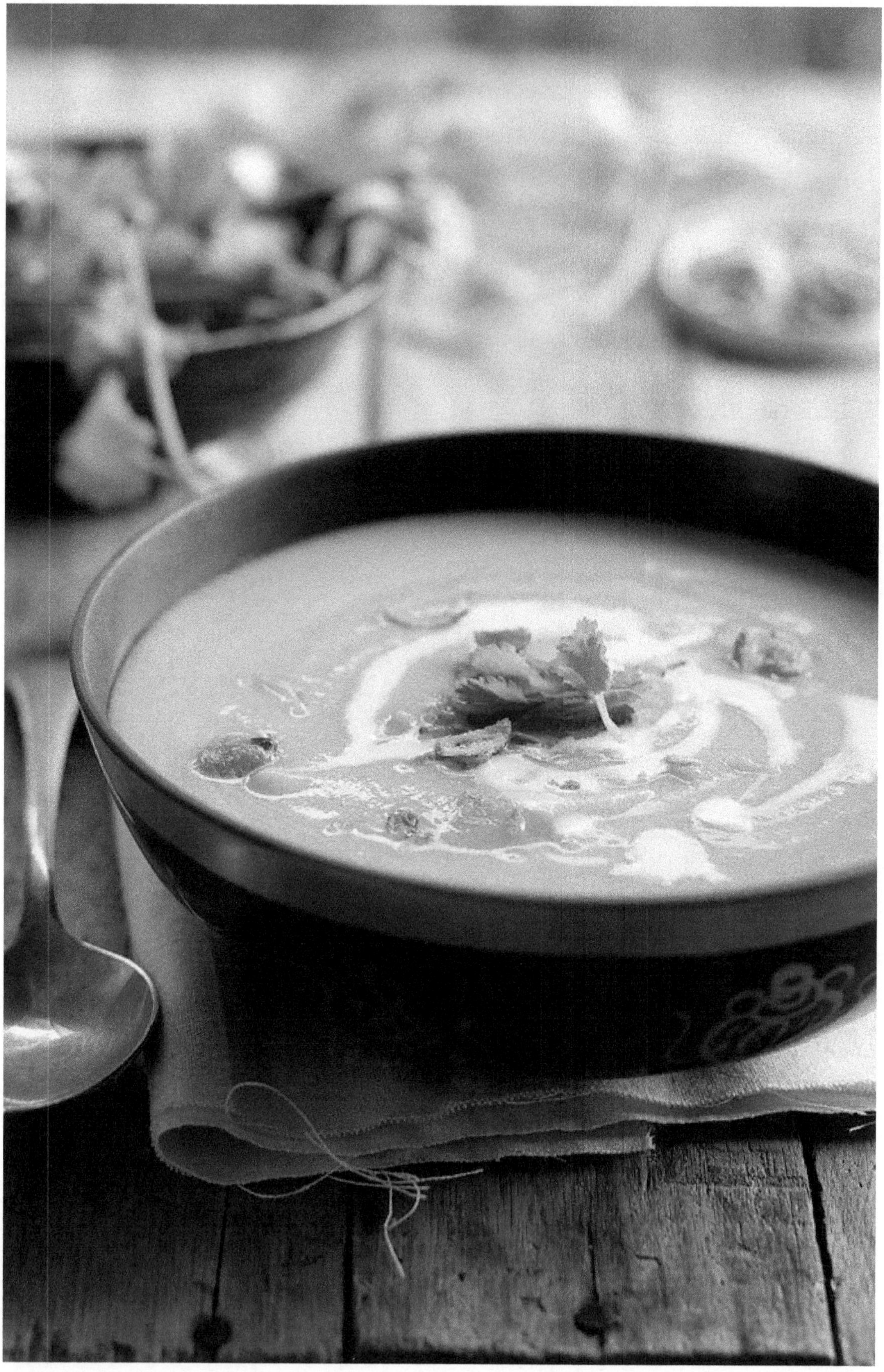

17 Buffalo Soup

(Ready in about 30 minutes | Serving 6 | Difficulty: Easy)

Per serving: Kcal 270, Fat: 16g, Net Carbs: 4g, Protein: 27g

Ingredients

- 1/2 large diced Onion
- 1 tbsp Olive oil
- 1/2 cup diced Celery
- 1 lb cooked shredded chicken
- 4 minced cloves Garlic
- 4 cups of Chicken broth
- 6 oz cubed Cream cheese
- 3 tbsp of Buffalo sauce
- 1/2 cup of half & half

Instructions

Select sauté setting on the instant pot. Add celery, onion and oil. Cook for around 10 minutes. Add garlic and sauté for around one minute. Turn the pot off and add chicken, buffalo sauce and broth. Cover the pot and seal it. Select soup setting and adjust the timer to 5 minutes. After done, release pressure naturally for around 5 minutes and turn to instant release and take the lid off. Ladle around a cup of liquid from the pot and add to the blender without chicken. Add cream cheese and puree. Pour mixture into the pot and add half and half and stir.

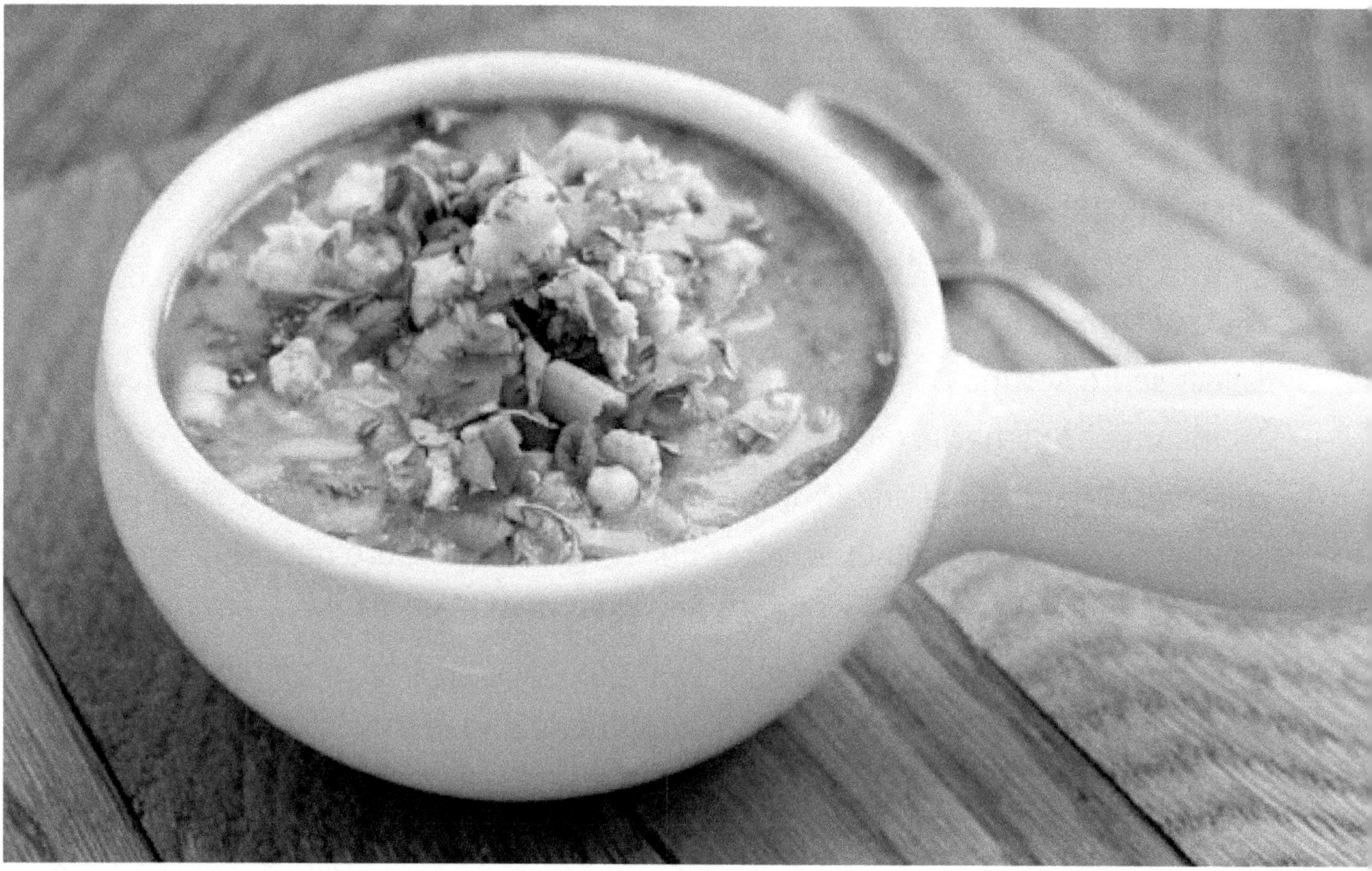

18 Jalapeno Soup

(Ready in about 25minutes | Serving 4 | Difficulty: Easy)

Per serving: Kcal 446, Fat: 35g, Net Carbs: 4g, Protein: 28g

Ingredients

- 4 slices of bacon
- 1/2 diced medium onion
- 2 tbsp of butter
- 1/4 cup chopped pickled jalapenos
- 2 cups shredded chicken cooked
- 2 cups of chicken broth
- 4 ounces of cream cheese
- Pepper and salt
- 1 cup sharp cheddar shredded
- 1/3 cup of heavy cream
- 1/4 tsp of garlic powder

Instructions

Fry bacon in a pan until crispy and crumble it and place aside. In the meantime, place the pot over moderate flame and add onion and butter. Saute for around 2 minutes and add half amount of bacon and jalapenos. Add chicken and broth and boil. Then reduce the flame and simmer for around 20 minutes. Add cream cheese to a bowl and microwave for around 20 seconds. Stir and add to soup. Mix heavy cream as well. Add grated cheese and until it is melted, stir. Serve with the rest of the bacon on top.

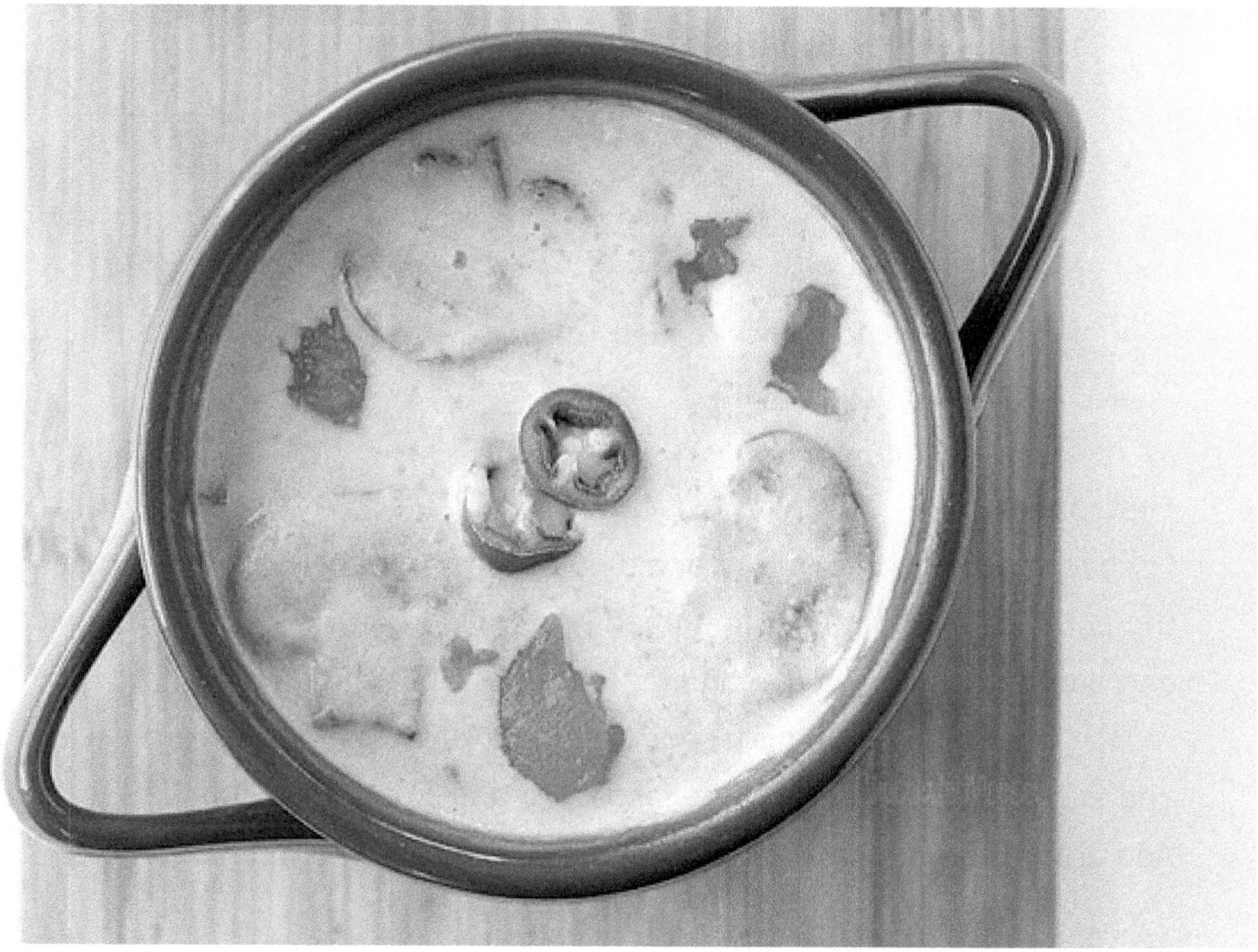

19 Sausage with Peppers

(Ready in about 2 hours 5 minutes | Serving 6 | Difficulty: Hard)

Per serving: Kcal 313, Fat: 21.7g, Net Carbs: 14g, Protein: 16.4g

Ingredients

- 1 tbsp Olive oil
- 3 diced into strips Bell peppers
- 6 medium Pork links of sausages
- 1 sliced large Onion
- 1/2 tsp of Sea salt
- 1 tbsp of Italian seasoning
- 6 minced cloves Garlic
- 1/4 tsp of Black pepper
- 1 1/2 cups of Marinara sauce

Instructions

Warm oil in a pan over moderate flame. Add sausage and cook for around 2 minutes on each side. Add the rest of the ingredients except marinara in the meantime in a slow cooker. Toss to mix and spread the marinara sauce in a layer on veggies. Add sausage and cook for around 3 hours on a high setting.

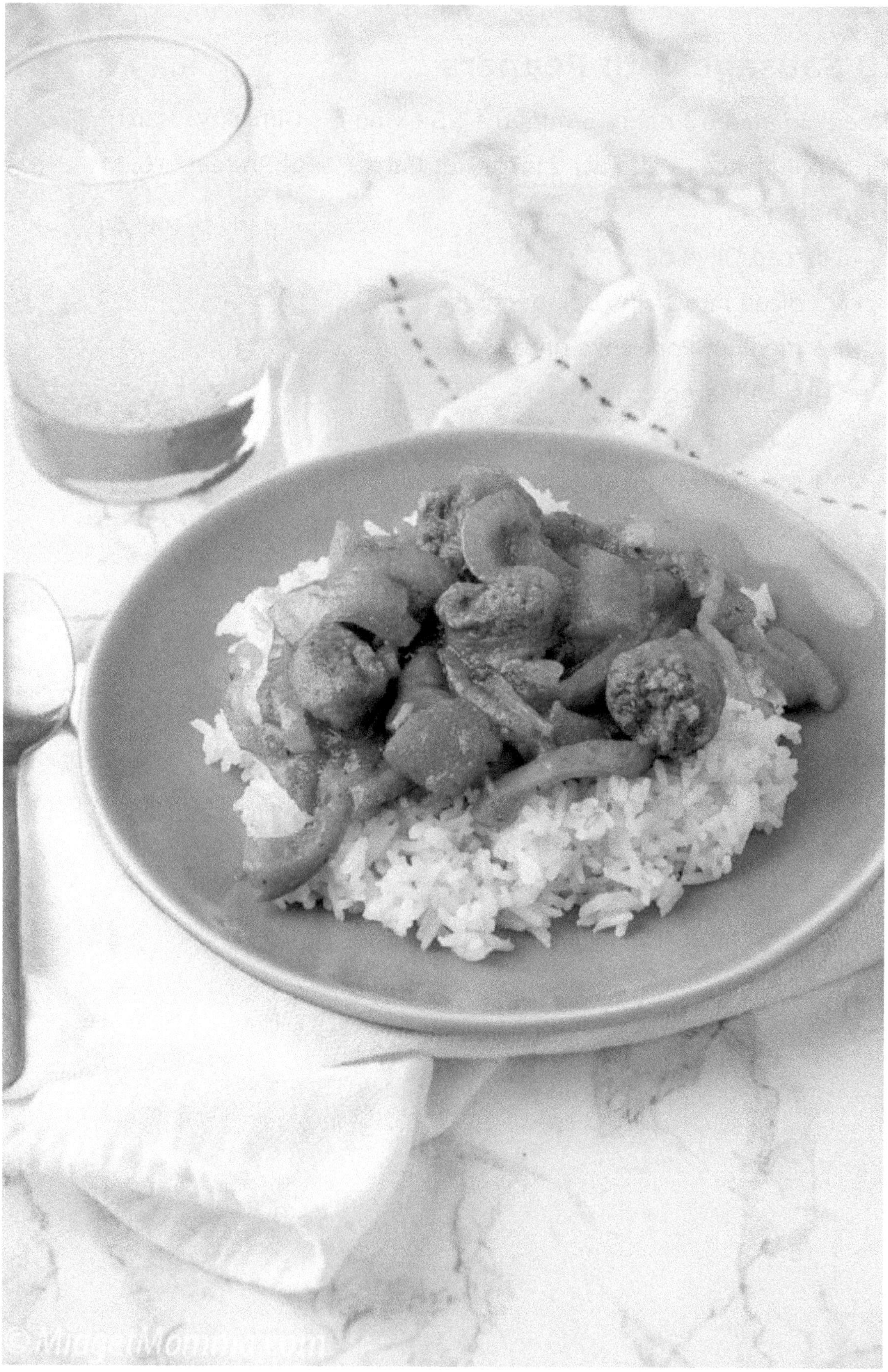
© MidgetMomma.com

20 Beef Barbacoa

(Ready in about 4 hours 10 minutes | Serving 9 | Difficulty: Hard)

Per serving: Kcal 242, Fat: 11g, Net Carbs: 2g, Protein: 32g

Ingredients

- 3 lb trimmed Beef brisket diced into chunks of 2 inch
- 2 Chipotle chiles in adobo medium
- 2 whole Bay leaf
- 1/2 cup of Beef broth
- 5 minced Garlic cloves
- 1 tbsp of Dried oregano
- 2 tbsp of Apple vinegar
- 2 tsp of Sea salt
- 2 tbsp of Lime juice
- 2 tsp of Cumin
- 1 tsp of Black pepper

Instructions

Add all the ingredients except beef plus bay leaves in a blender and puree. You will get a smooth mixture. Add beef to the slow cooker and pour blender mixture on it. Add bay leaves and cook for 6 hours at the high setting.

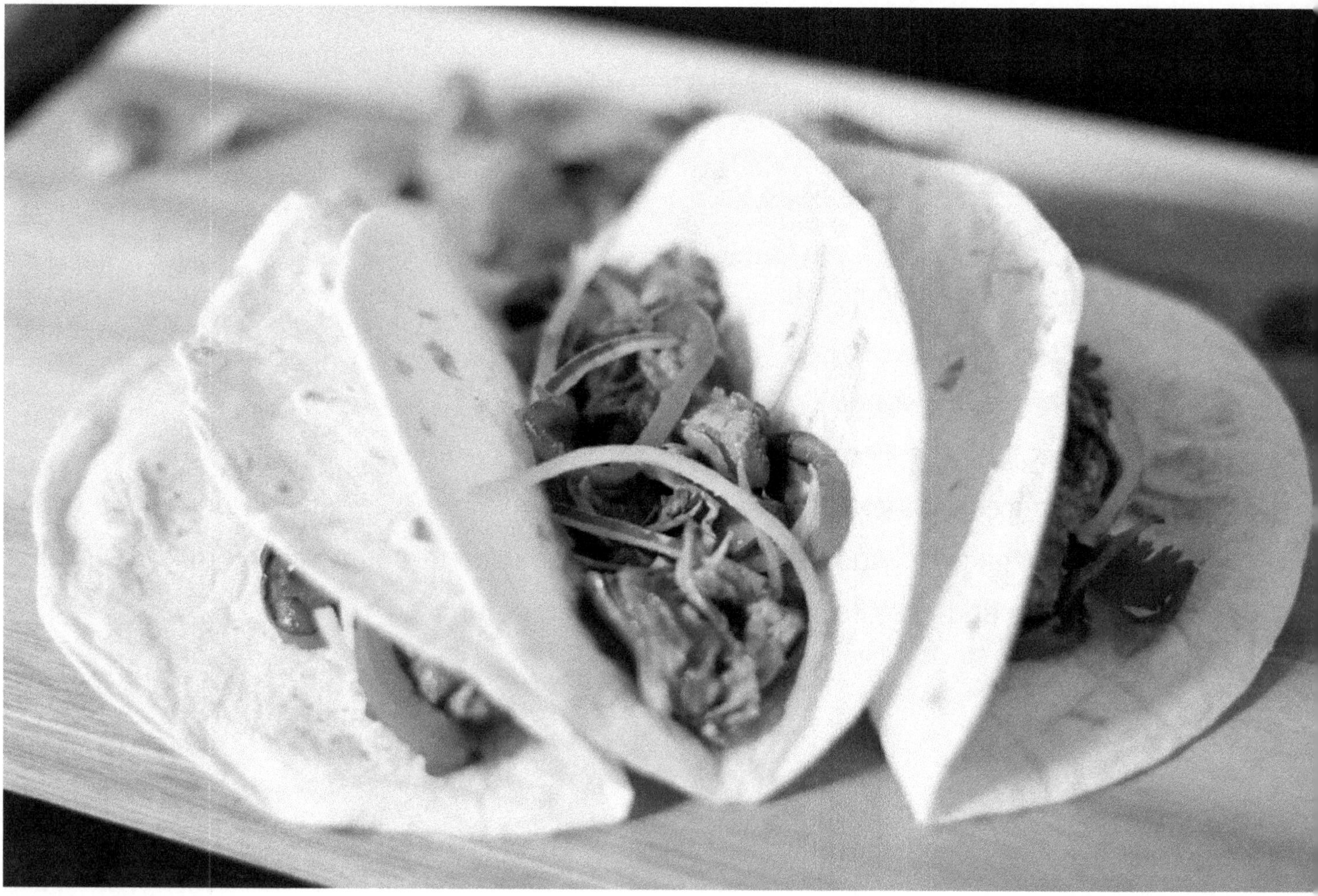

21 Cauliflower Shrimp

(Ready in about 30 minutes | Serving 2 | Difficulty: Easy)

Per serving: Kcal 302, Fat: 18g, Net Carbs: 13g, Protein: 24g

Spicy Shrimp

- 1 tbsp of paprika
- 1 pound deveined shrimp peeled
- 2 tsp of garlic powder
- 1 tbsp of olive oil
- 1/2tsp of cayenne pepper
- Black pepper ground and salt

Cauliflower Grits

- 1 tbsp of unsalted butter
- 1 cup of whole milk
- 4 cups of riced cauliflower
- 1/2 cup of crumbled goat cheese
- Black pepper ground and salt

Garlic Arugula

- 1 tbsp of extra-virgin olive oil
- 4 cups of baby arugula
- 3 sliced garlic cloves
- Black pepper ground and salt

Instructions

Mix cayenne, paprika and garlic powder in a bowl. Add shrimp to a sealable bag and add the mixture in it. Toss and refrigerate the bag. Melt butter in a pot over moderate flame. Cook cauliflower rice for around 3minutes. Add half amount of milk and simmer for around 8 minutes. Add rest of milk and simmer for around 10 minutes. Add goat cheese and season using pepper and salt. Warm 1 tbsp oil in a pan for garlic arugula. Sauté garlic for around 1 minute. Add arugula and sauté for around 4minutes. Season using pepper and salt and take out on a plate. Add the rest of the olive oil in this pan and sauté shrimp for around 5 minutes. Season using pepper and salt. Divide grits equally among 4 plates and top with a quarter amount of each shrimp and arugula.

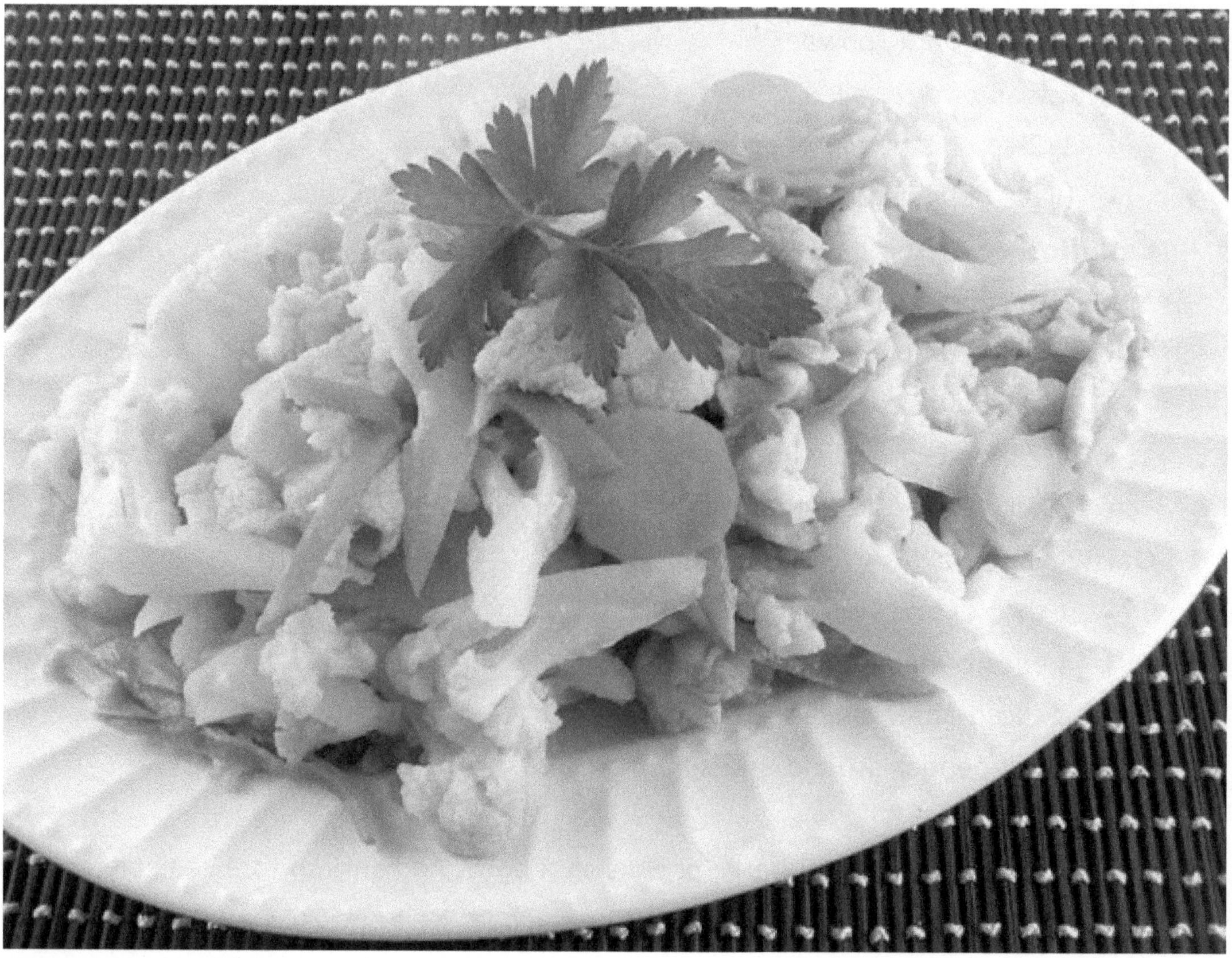

22 Cheese Spinach

(Ready in about 10 minutes | Serving 4 | Difficulty: Easy)

Per serving: Kcal 166, Fat: 15.1, Net Carbs: 1.7, Protein: 4.4

Ingredients

- 1 tbsp butter, room temperature
- 1 clove garlic, minced
- 10 ounces spinach
- 1/2 tsp garlic salt
- 1/4 tsp ground black pepper, or more to taste
- 1/2tsp cayenne pepper
- 3 ounces cream cheese
- 1/2 cup double cream

Instructions

Add butter to a pan and melt over moderate flame. Cook garlic for around 30 seconds and add spinach. Cook for around 2 minutes, covered. Season with cayenne, pepper and salt. Add cream and cheese and cook until it melts.

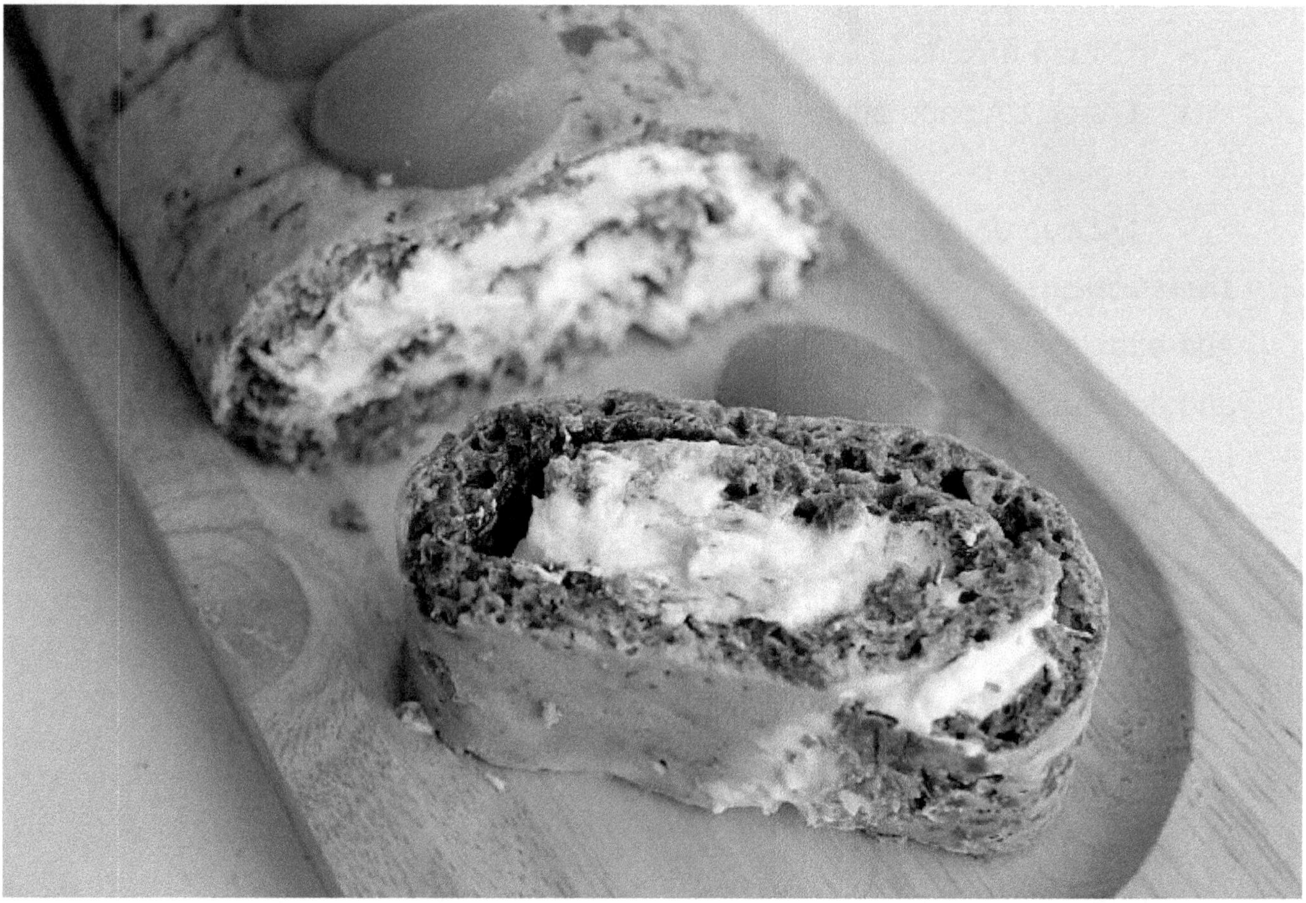

23 Tangy Chicken Drumettes

(Ready in about 40 minutes | Serving 4 | Difficulty: Moderate)

Per serving: Kcal 209, Fat: 12.2g, Net Carbs: 0.4, Protein: 23.2g

Ingredients

- 1 pound chicken drumettes
- 1 tbsp olive oil
- 2 tbsp butter, melted
- 1garlic cloves, sliced
- Fresh juice of 1/2 lemon
- 2 tbsp white wine
- Salt and ground black pepper, to taste
- 1 tbsp fresh scallions, chopped

Instructions

Preheat the oven to 440 degrees F. Line a pan using parchment paper and add chicken. Drizzle with butter and oil. Add the rest of the ingredients and bake for around 35 minutes. Garnish with scallions.

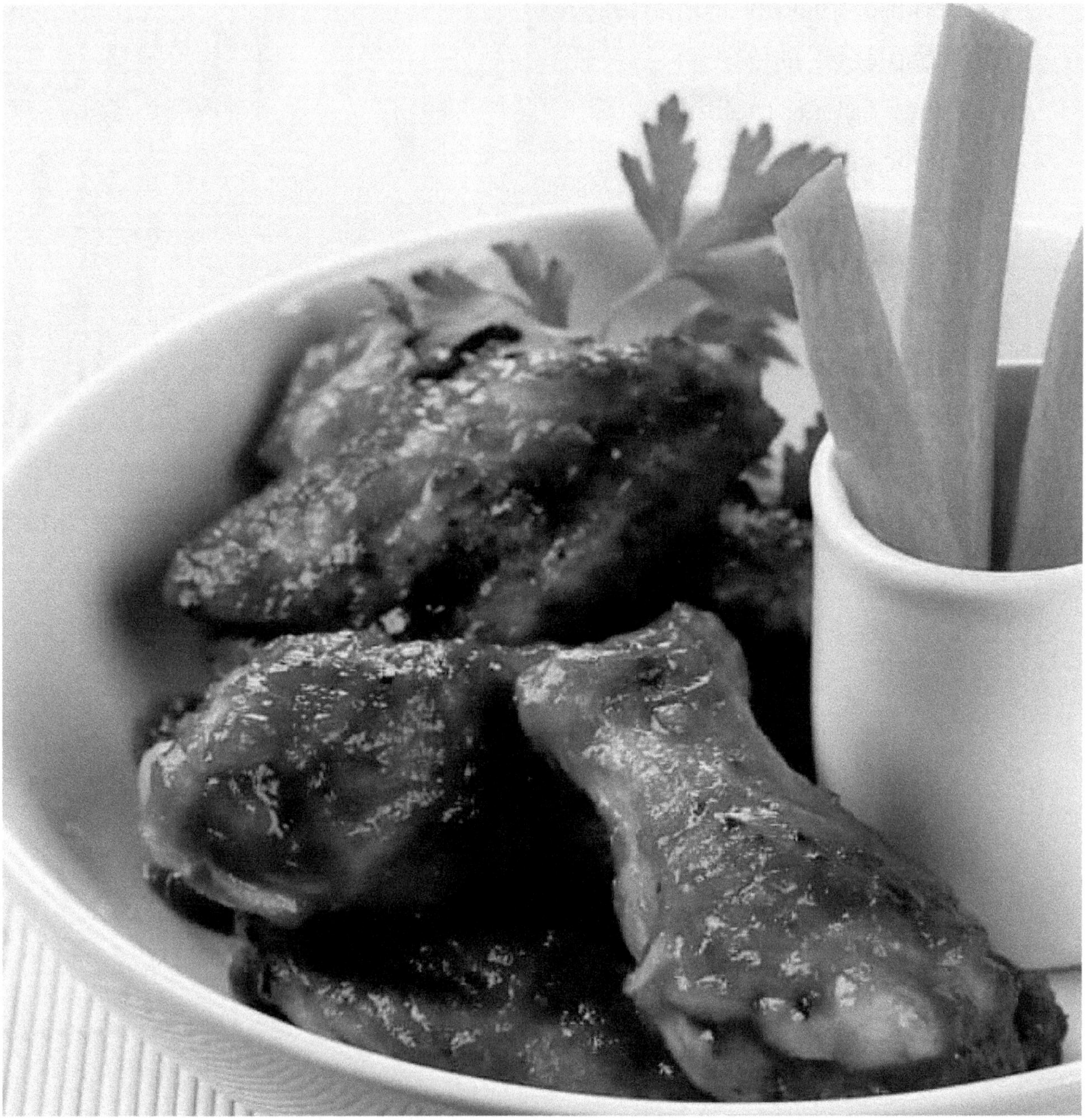

24 Ranch Chicken

(Ready in about 20 minutes | Serving 4 | Difficulty: Easy)

Per serving: Kcal 295, Fat: 19.5g, Net Carbs: 2.9g, Protein: 3.1g

Ingredients

- 2 chicken breasts
- 2 tbsp butter, melted
- 1 tsp salt
- 1/2 tsp garlic powder
- 1/2 tsp cayenne pepper
- 1/2 tsp black peppercorns, crushed
- 1/2 tbsp ranch seasoning mix
- 4 ounces Ricotta cheese, room temperature
- 1/2 cup Monterey-Jack cheese, grated
- 4 slices bacon, chopped
- 1/4 cup scallions, chopped

Instructions

Preheat the oven to 370 degrees F. Drizzle butter over chicken. Add seasonings to chicken and cook chicken in the pan for around 5 minutes on each side. Coat a baking dish and add chicken. Add bacon and cheese and bake for around 12 minutes. Add scallions on top.

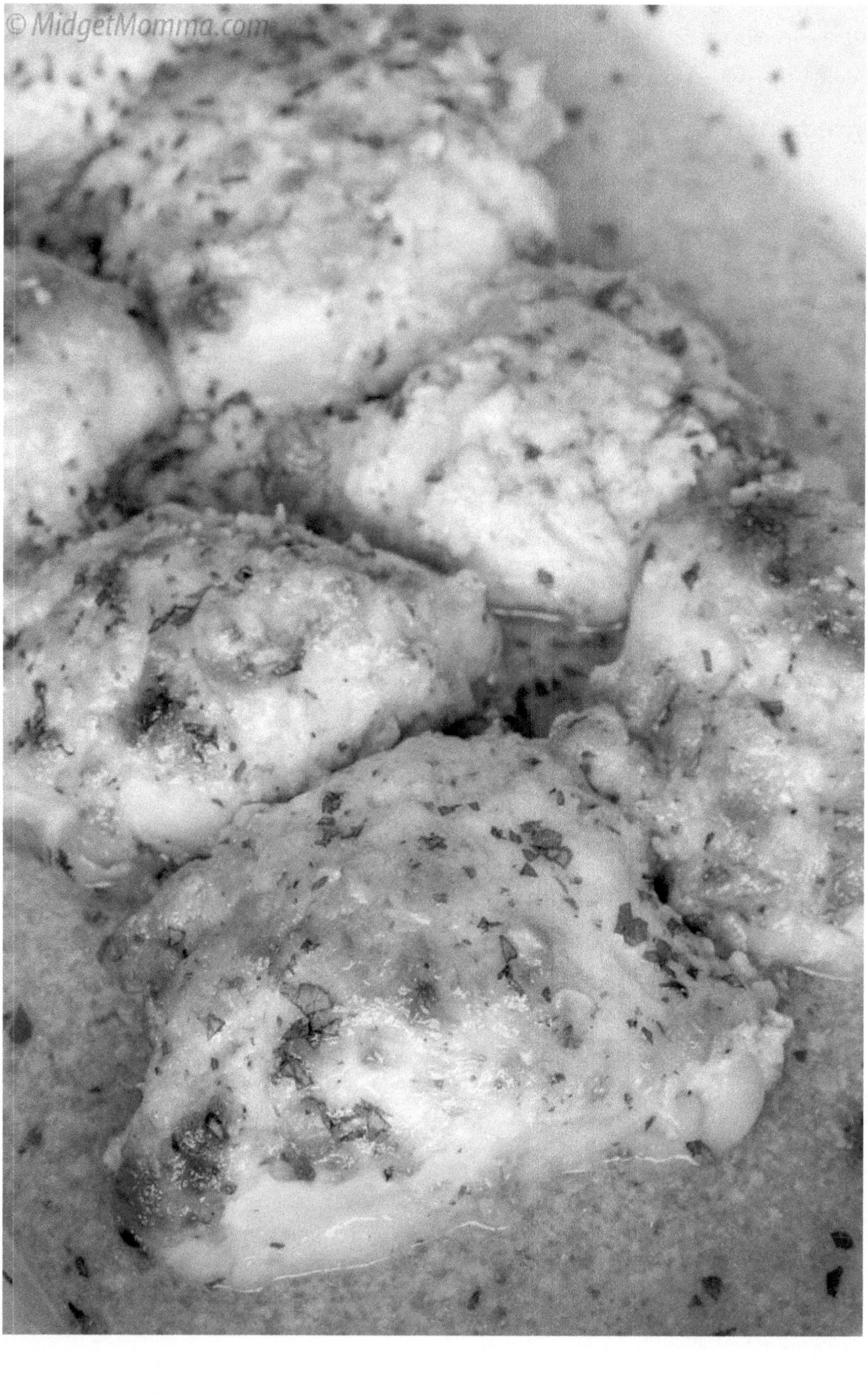
© MidgetMomma.com

25 Garlic Chicken Wings

(Ready in about 25 minutes | Serving 4 | Difficulty: Easy)

Per serving: Kcal 131, Fat: 7.8g, Net Carbs: 1.8g, Protein: 13.4g

Ingredients

- 8 chicken wings
- 2 tbsp ghee, melted

The Marinade

- 2 garlic cloves, minced
- 1/4 cup leeks, chopped
- 2 tbsp lemon juice
- Salt and ground black pepper, to taste
- 1/2 tsp paprika
- 1 tsp dried rosemary

Instructions

Add marinade ingredients in a bowl and coat chicken with it. Cover and leave for around1 an hour. Preheat the grill to moderate temperature. Drizzle chicken with melted ghee and grill for around 20 minutes.

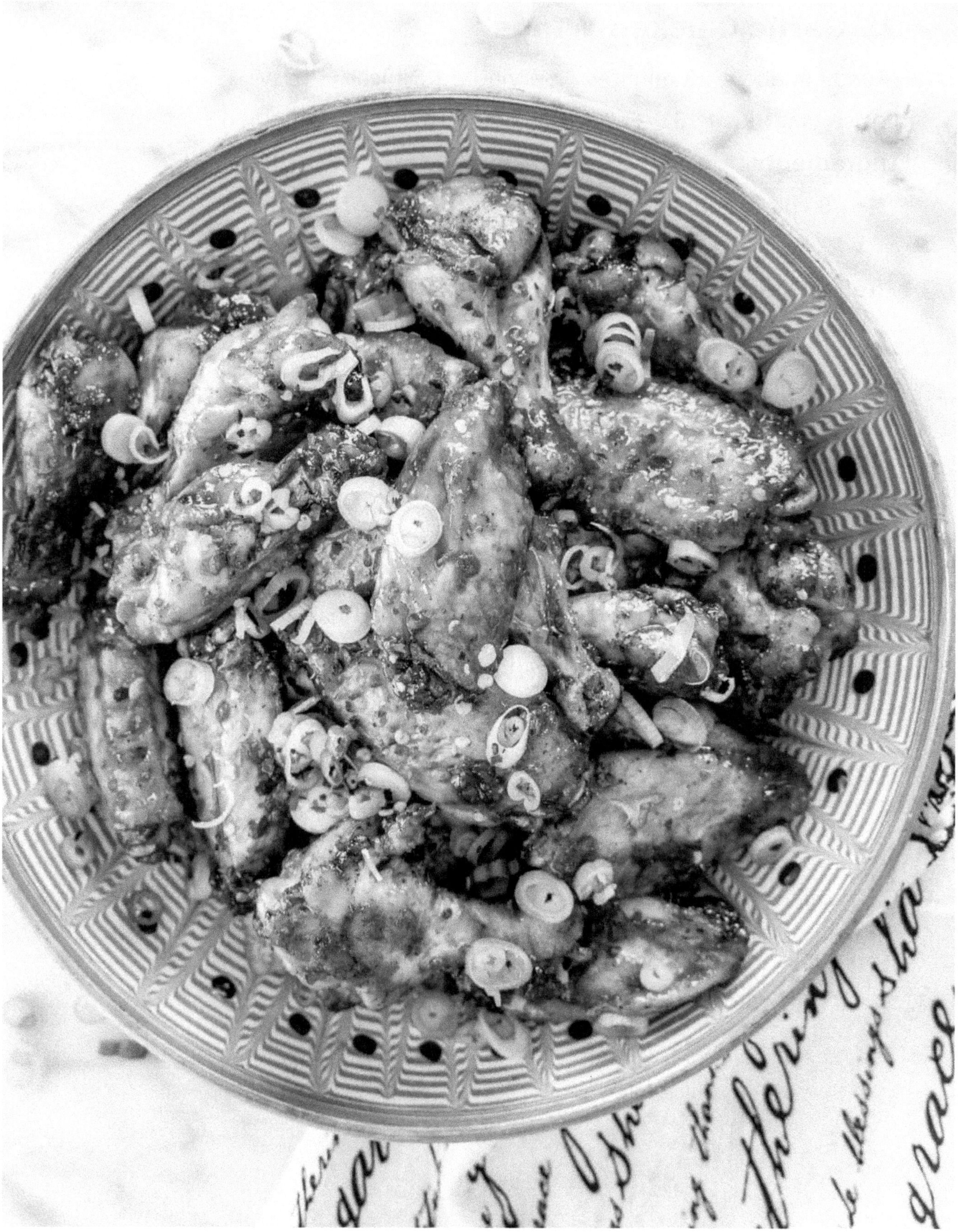

26 Steak Salad

(Ready in about 20 minutes | Serving 4 | Difficulty: Easy)

Per serving: Kcal 231, Fat: 17g, Net Carbs: 6g, Protein: 13.8g

Ingredients

- 2 tbsp olive oil
- 8 ounces flank steak, salt-and-pepper-seasoned
- 1cucumber, sliced
- 1/2 cup onions, finely sliced
- 1 ripe avocado, peeled and sliced
- 2 medium-sized heirloom tomatoes, sliced
- 2 ounces baby arugula
- 1 tbsp fresh coriander, chopped
- 3 tbsp lime juice

Instructions

Warm 1 tbsp oil in a pan over moderate flame and cook steak for around 5 minutes. Transfer steak to bowl and add rest of ingredients. Drizzle the rest of the oil and lime juice and eat after chilling.

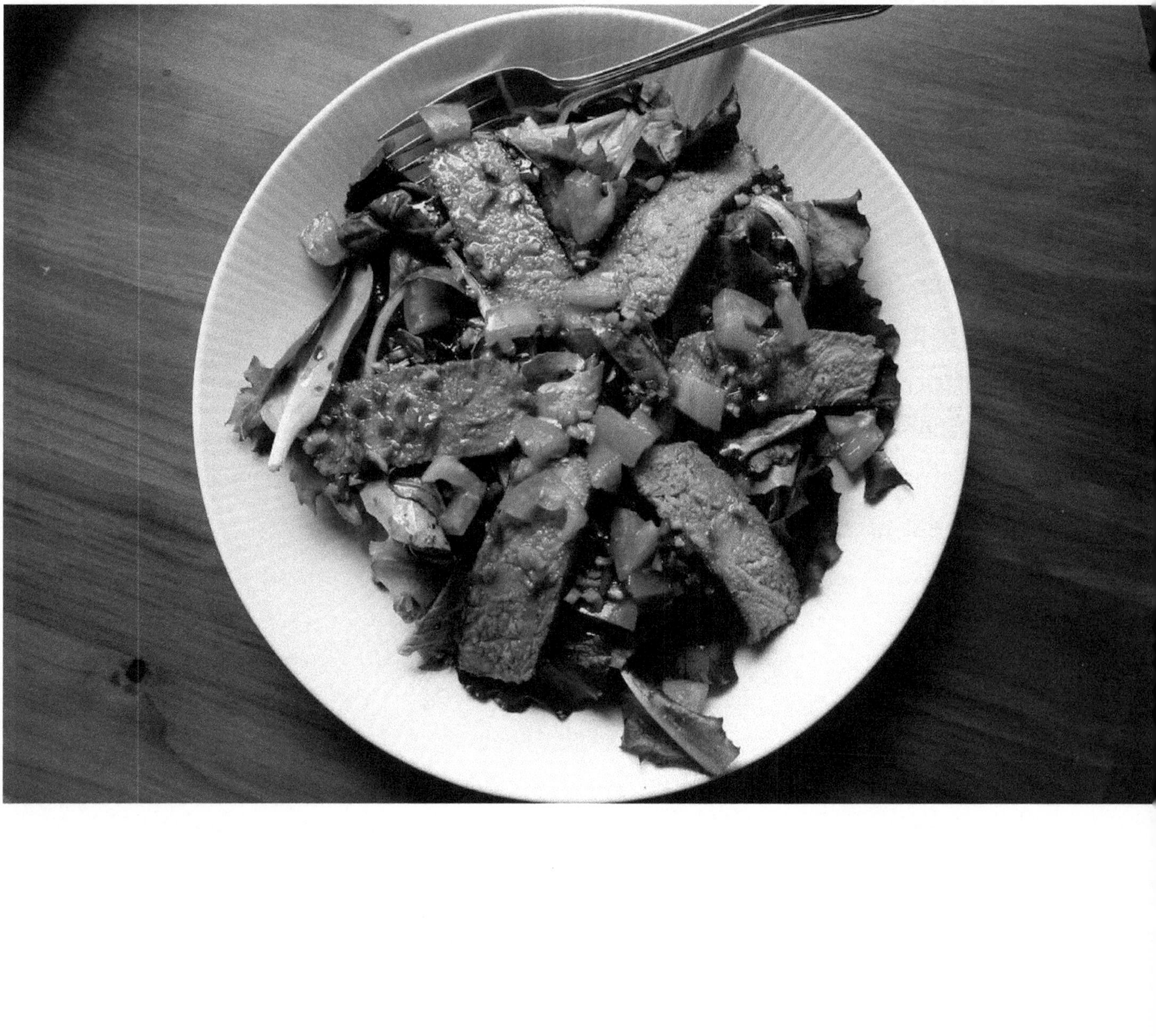

27 Catfish

(Ready in about 25 minutes | Serving 4 | Difficulty: Easy)

Per serving: Kcal 510, Fat: 40g, Net Carbs: 5.5g, Protein: 31.3g

Ingredients

- 1 tbsp of sesame oil
- 4 scallions
- 11 ounces of cauliflower
- 2 ounces of butter
- 1 minced garlic clove
- Black pepper ground and salt
- 1 tspgrated ginger root
- Cayenne pepper
- 1 sprig crushed rosemary
- 2 sprigs crushed dried thyme
- 24 ounces of catfish
- 1/2 cup of double cream
- 1/2 cup of cream cheese
- 1 egg

Instructions

Preheat the oven to around 390 degrees F. Spray casserole dish using cooking spray. Add oil to pan and warm over moderate flame. Cook scallions and cauliflower for around 5 minutes. Add ginger and garlic and cook for one more minute. Transfer veggies to the dish and sprinkle using seasonings. Top with catfish. Mix cream, cheese and egg in a bowl and spread over casserole. Add butter slices on top and bake for around 22 minutes.

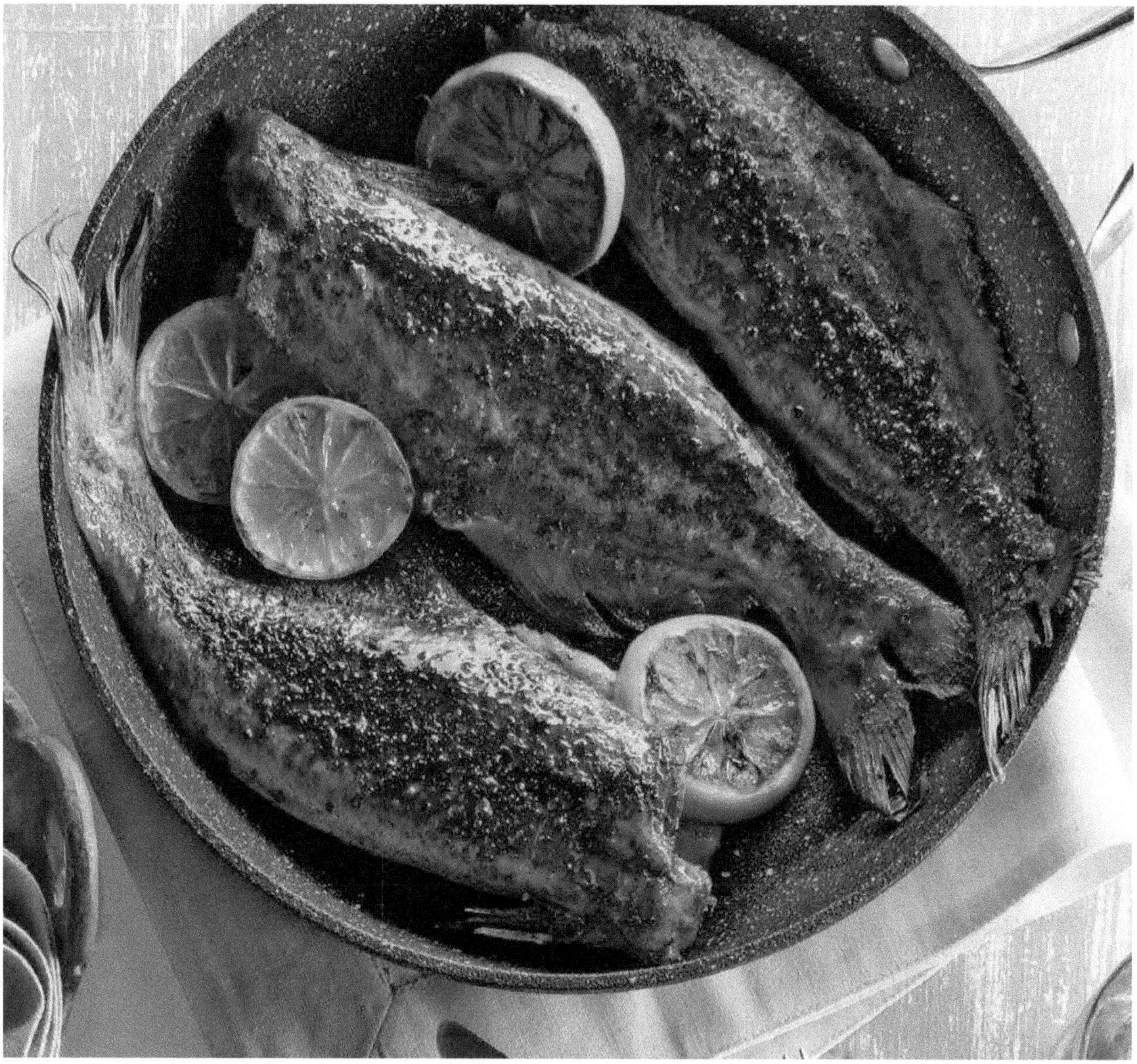

28 Salad- Swedish Style

(Ready in about 8 minutes | Serving 3 | Difficulty: Easy)

Per serving: Kcal 134, Fat: 7.9g, Net Carbs: 5.4g, Protein: 10.2g

Ingredients

- 1/2 cup of baby spinach
- 6 ounces of flaked herring pieces pickled
- 2tbspof basil leaves
- 1 chopped bell pepper
- 2 tbspof chopped fresh chives
- Black pepper ground and salt
- 1 tsp of minced garlic
- 1 chopped red onion
- 2 tbspof freshly squeezed lime juice

Instructions

Add veggies to a bowl and mix. Drizzle lime juice and sprinkle using pepper and salt. Toss and enjoy your salad.

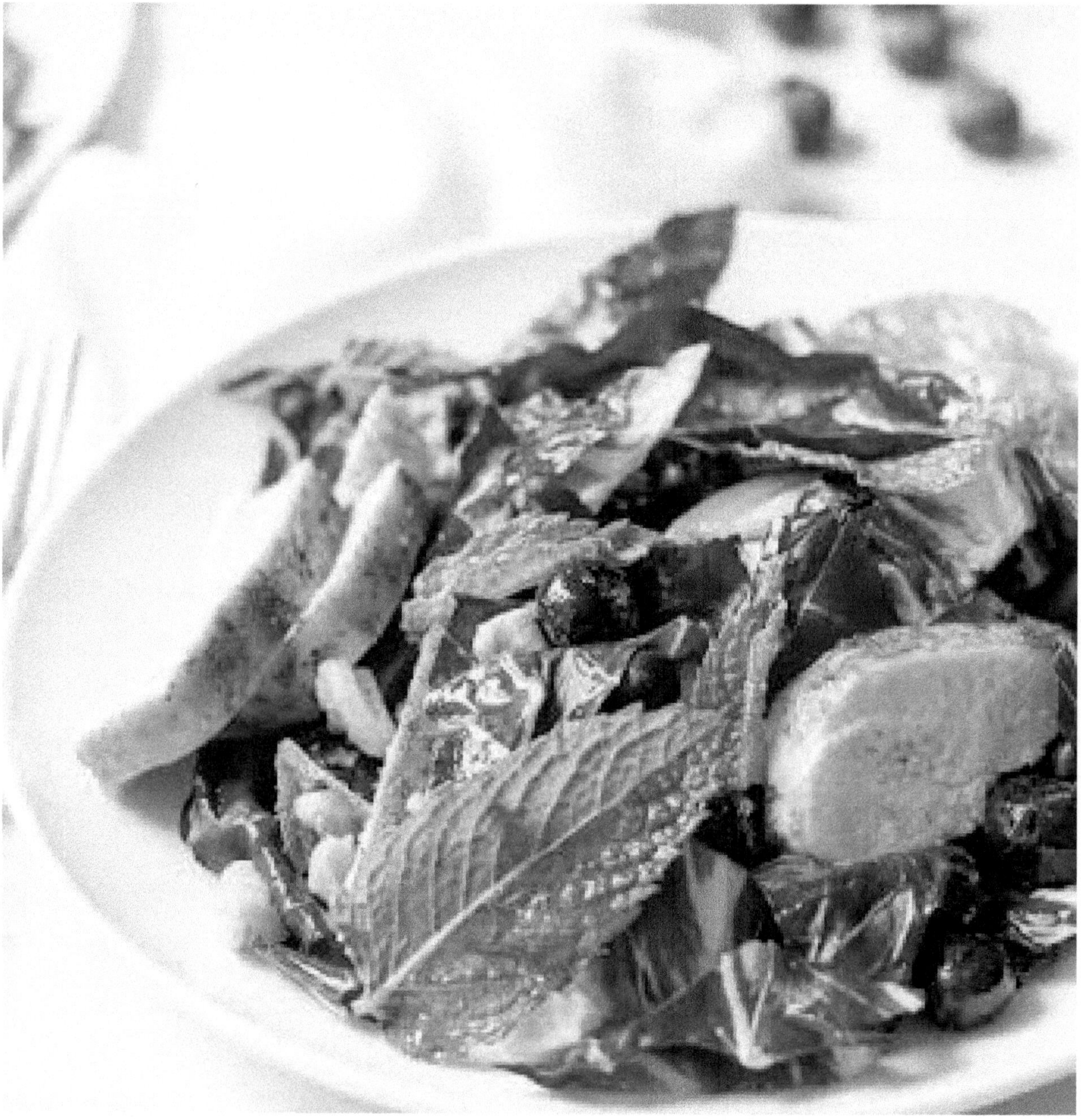

29 Fish Medley

(Ready in about 20 minutes | Serving 4 | Difficulty: Easy)

Per serving: Kcal 151, Fat: 3g, Net Carbs: 5.8, Protein: 24.4g

Ingredients

- 1 tsp sesame oil
- 1/2 cup scallions, thinly sliced
- 1/2 tsp fresh ginger, grated
- 1/2 tsp garlic, crushed
- 1 tsp red curry paste
- 2 whole star anise
- 1 tsp smoked paprika
- 2 ripe tomatoes, crushed
- Ground black pepper and sea salt
- 1 pound snapper, cut into bite-sized pieces

Instructions

Add oil to a pot and warm over moderate flame. Add ginger and scallions and cook for around 1 minute. Add the rest of the ingredients and reduce the flame. Simmer for around 15 minutes and enjoy.

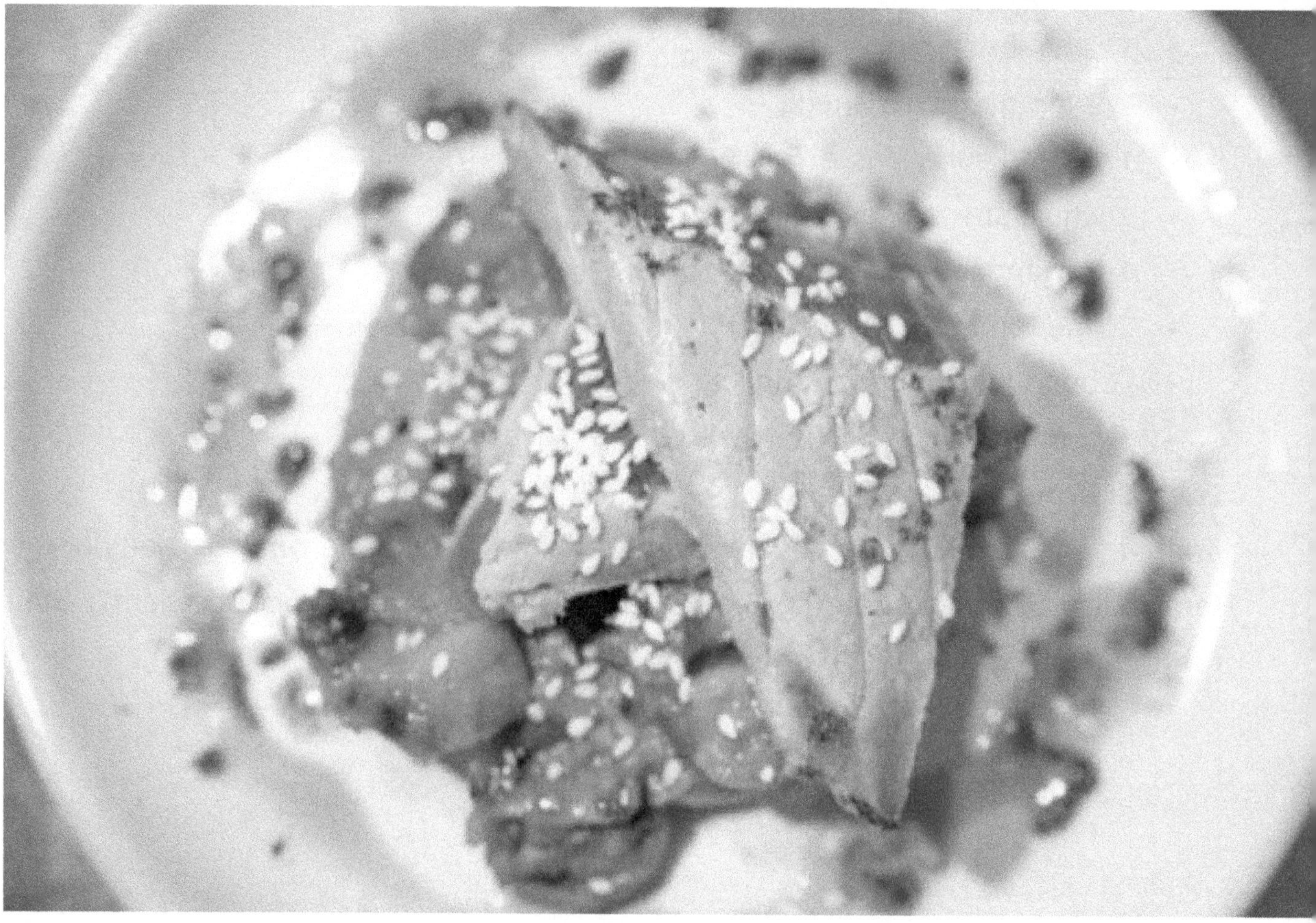

30 Ham Wraps

(Ready in about 10 minutes | Serving 3 | Difficulty: Easy)

Per serving: Kcal 308, Fat: 19.9g, Net Carbs: 4.3g, Protein: 27.8g

Ingredients

- 1/2 cup dry white wine
- 1/2 cup water
- 1/2 tsp mixed peppercorns
- 1/2 tsp dry mustard powder
- 1/2 pound ahi tuna steak
- 6 slices of ham
- 1/2Hass avocado, peeled, pitted and sliced
- 1 tbsp fresh lemon juice6 lettuce leaves

Instructions

Add all the ingredients except lemon and avocado in a bowl and mix. Add to pan with tuna and simmer for around 5 minutes on each side. Slice the tuna after removing the liquid. Drizzle lemon over and add avocado. Roll wraps and place on a lettuce leaf.

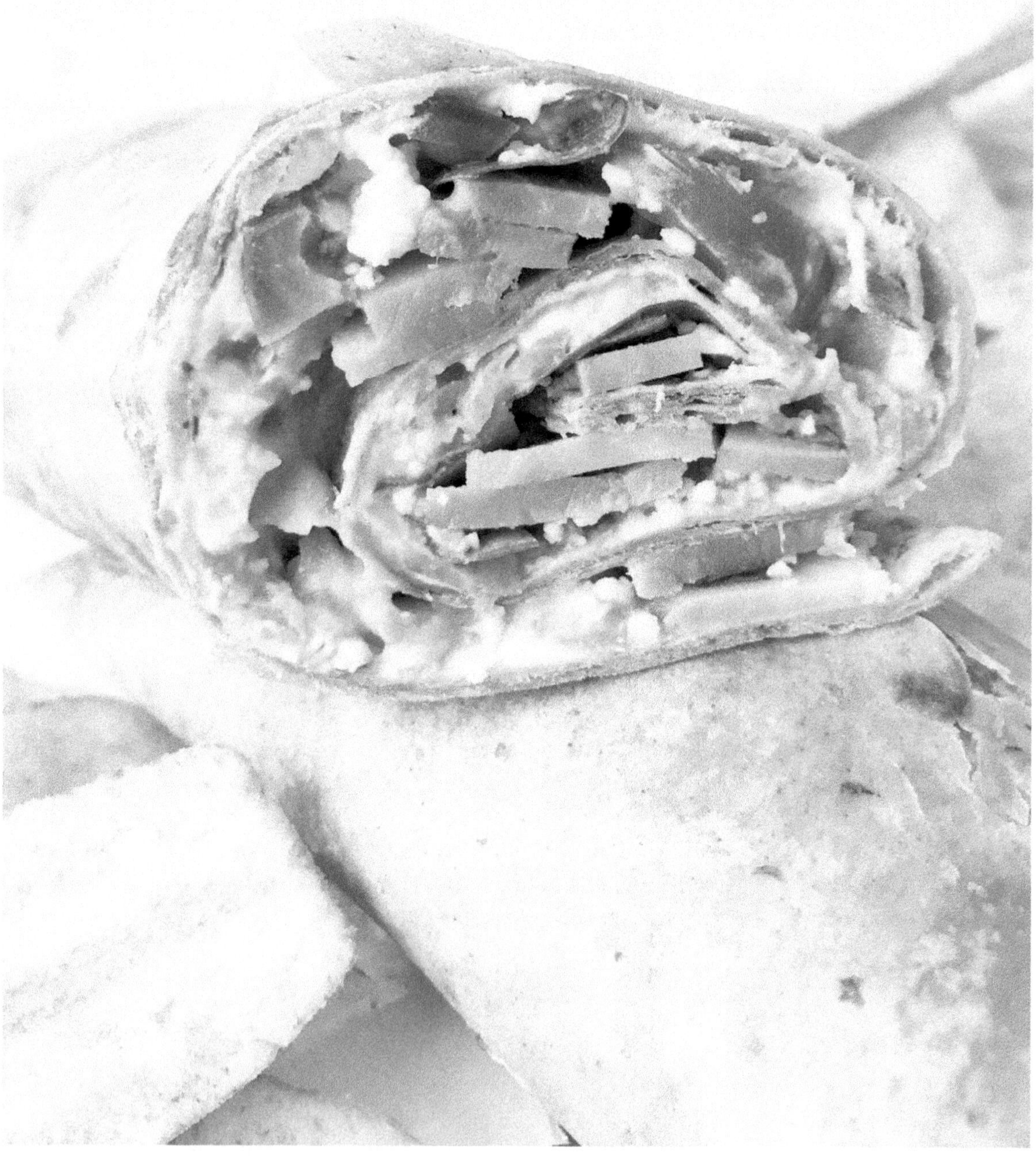

31 Alaskan Cod

(Ready in about 10 minutes | Serving 4 | Difficulty: Easy)

Per serving: Kcal 166, Fat: 8.2g, Net Carbs: 2.6g, Protein: 19.8g

Ingredients

- 1 tbsp coconut oil
- 4 Alaskan cod fillets
- Salt and freshly ground black pepper, to taste
- 6 leaves basil, chiffonade
- Mustard Cream Sauce:
- 1 tsp yellow mustard
- 1 tsp paprika
- 1/4 tsp ground bay leaf
- 3 tbsp cream cheese
- 1/2 cup Greek-style yogurt
- 1 garlic clove, minced
- 1 tsp lemon zest
- 1 tbsp fresh parsley, minced
- Sea salt and ground black pepper, to taste

Instructions

Add oil to the pan and warm over moderate flame. Add fish and sear for around 3 minutes on each side. Season using pepper and salt. Add sauce ingredients in a bowl and mix. Top fillets with sauce and garnish with basil leaves.

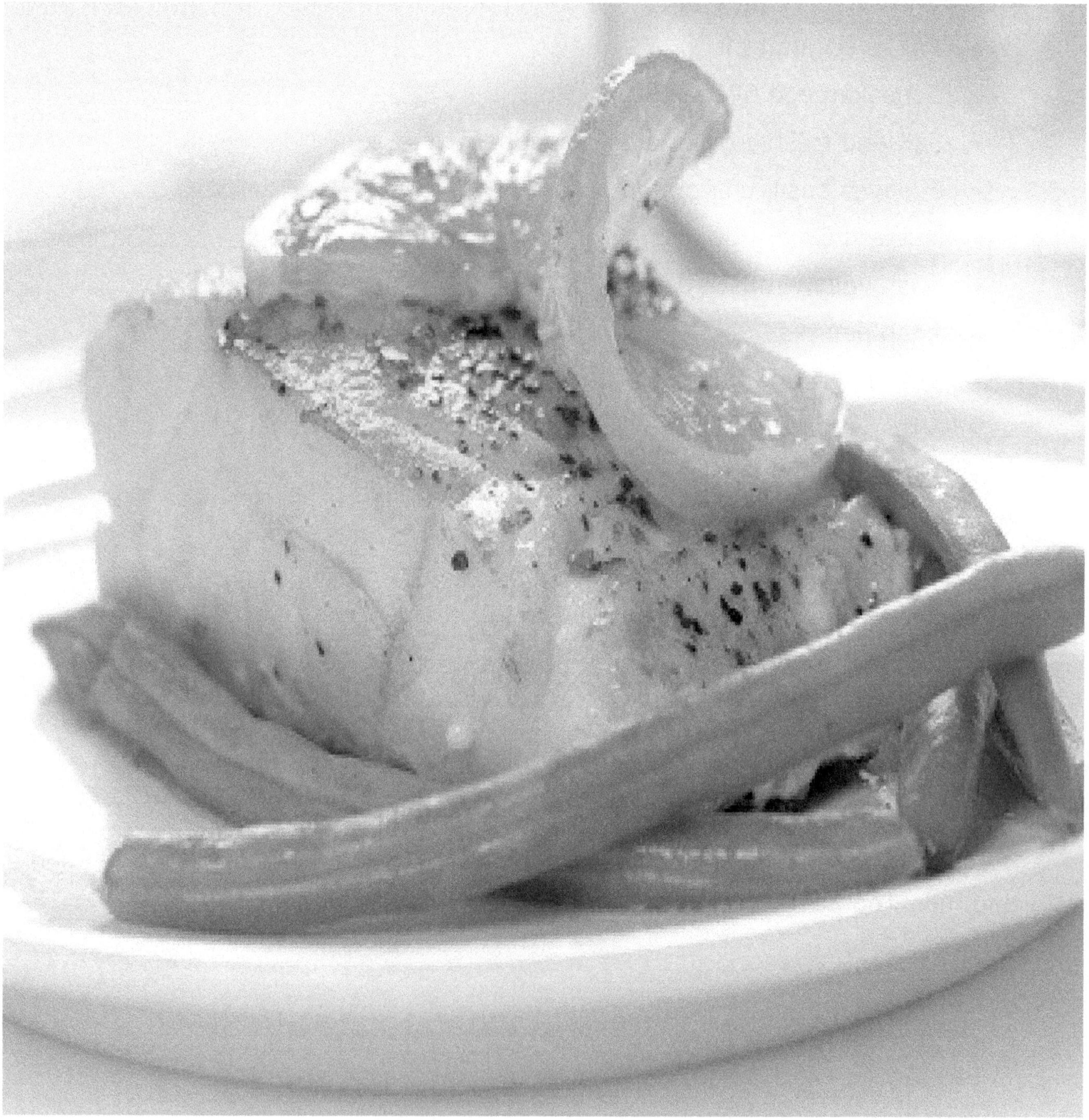

32 Paprika Omelet

(Ready in about 10 minutes | Serving 2 | Difficulty: Easy)

Per serving: Kcal 287, Fat: 22.6g, Net Carbs: 1.3g, Protein: 19.8g

Ingredients

- 2 tsp ghee, room temperature
- 4 eggs, whisked
- 4 tbsp goat cheese
- 1tsp paprika
- Sea salt and ground black pepper, to taste

Instructions

Add ghee to the pan and melt over moderate flame. Whisk eggs in a bowl and add to the pan. Cover the pan and reduce the flame to a low temperature. Cook for around 4 minutes. Add paprika and cheese and cook for 3 more minutes. Season using pepper and salt.

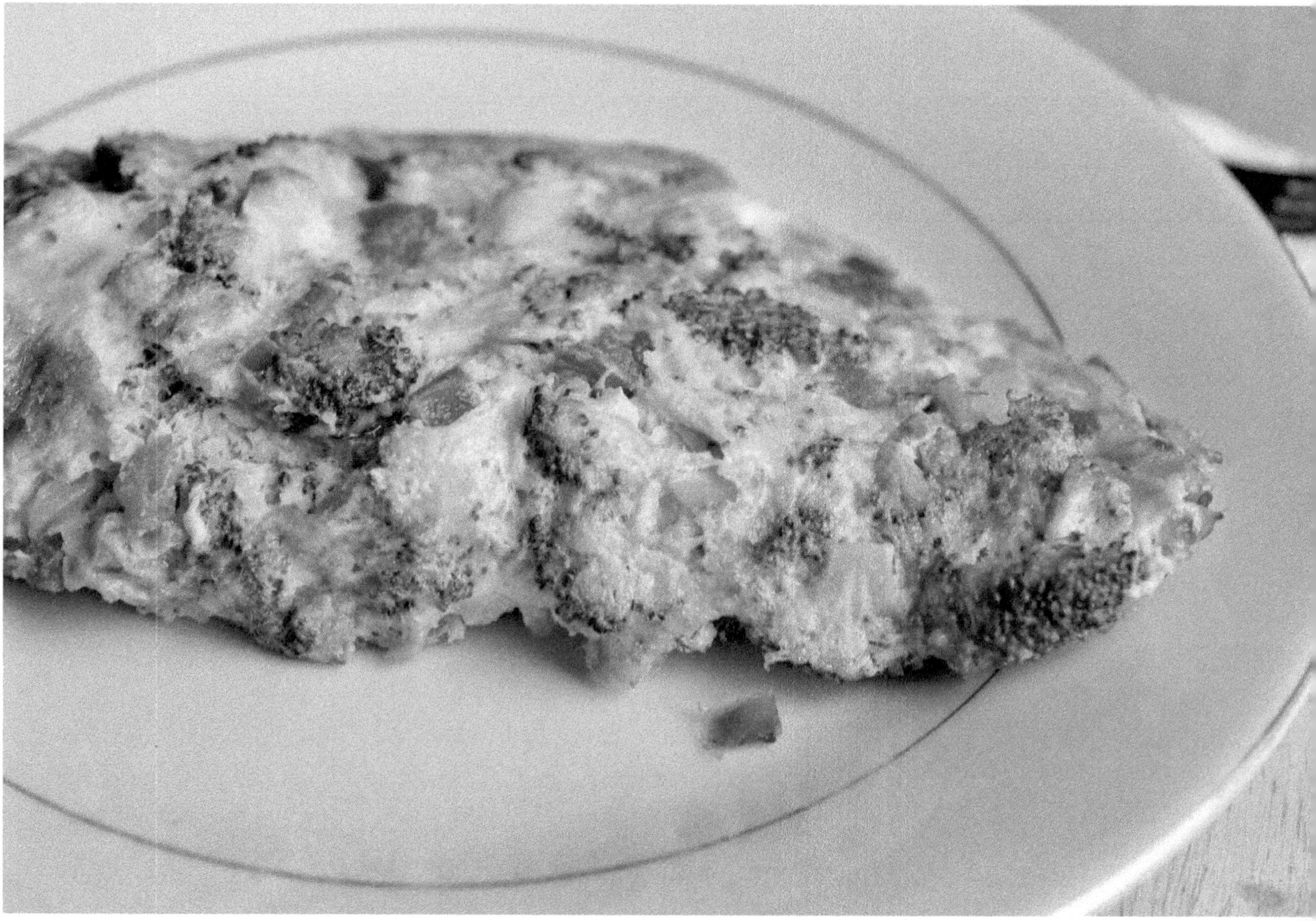

33 Boiled Eggs

(Ready in about 10 minutes | Serving 3 | Difficulty: Easy)

Per serving: Kcal 222, Fat: 17.6g, Net Carbs: 5.7g, Protein: 12.2

Ingredients

- 6 eggs
- 1/2 tsp kosher salt
- 1/2 tsp ground black pepper
- 1/2 tsp cayenne pepper
- 1/2 tsp dried dill weed
- 1 avocado, pitted and sliced
- 1tbsp lemon juice

Instructions

Add water to the pan and boil. Add eggs and cook for around 6 minutes on low heat. Peel eggs and cut them in half. Sprinkle with seasonings and drizzle lemon juice over avocado slices. Serve on the side with eggs.

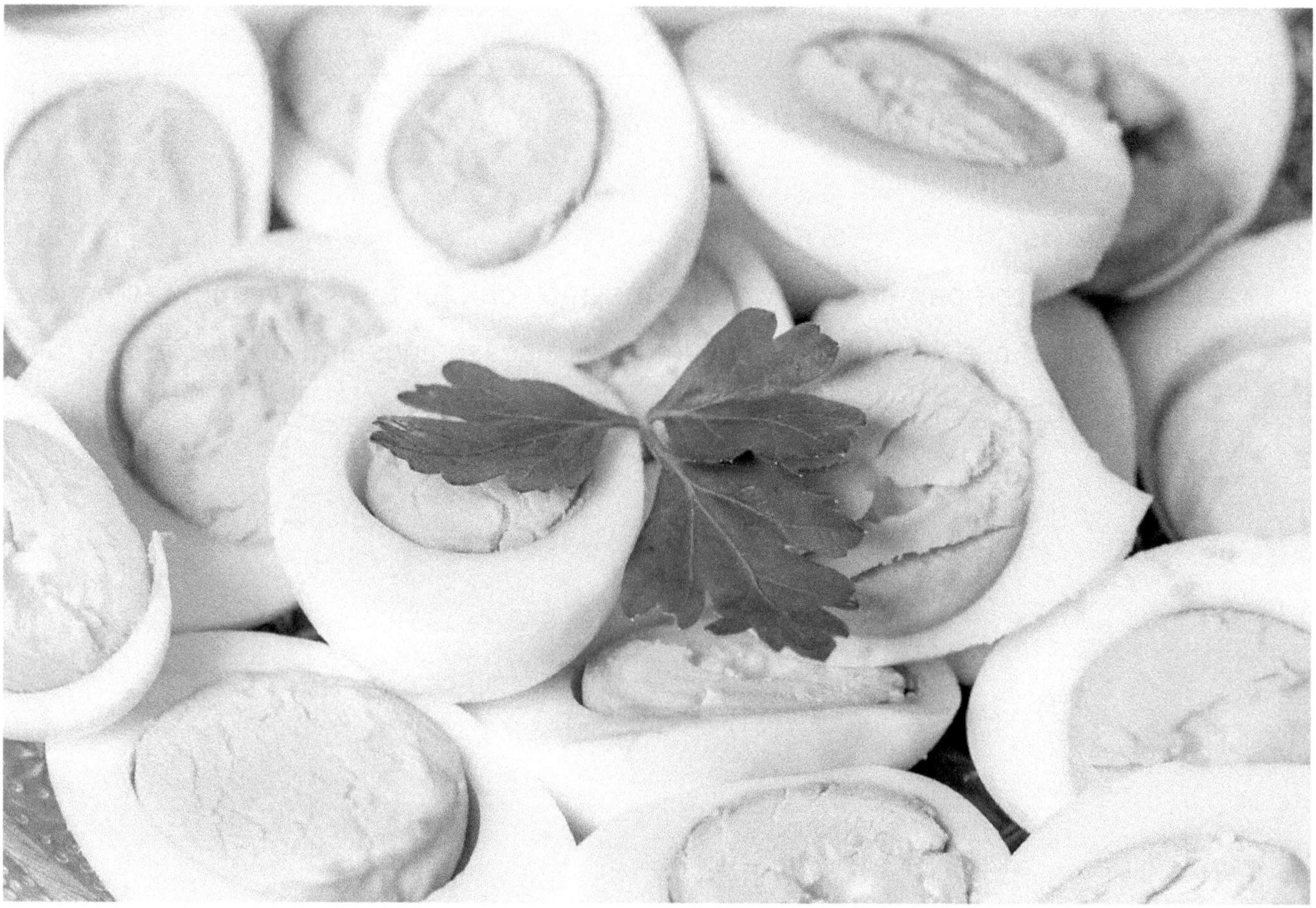

34 Stuffed Peppers

(Ready in about 45 minutes | Serving 3 | Difficulty: Moderate)

Per serving: Kcal 194, Fat: 13.9g, Net Carbs: 3.5g, Protein: 13.3

Ingredients

- 3 bell peppers, halved, seeds removed
- 3 eggs, whisked
- 1 cup Mexican cheese blend
- 1 tsp chili powder
- 1 garlic clove, minced
- 1 tsp onion powder
- 1ripe tomato, pureed
- 1 tsp mustard powder

Instructions

Preheat the oven to 370 degrees F. Add oil to the pan and combine eggs, chili powder, cheese, onion powder and garlic in a bowl. Divide filling equally among bell peppers. Mix mustard powder and tomatoes and pour in pan. Bake for around 40 minutes, covered with foil

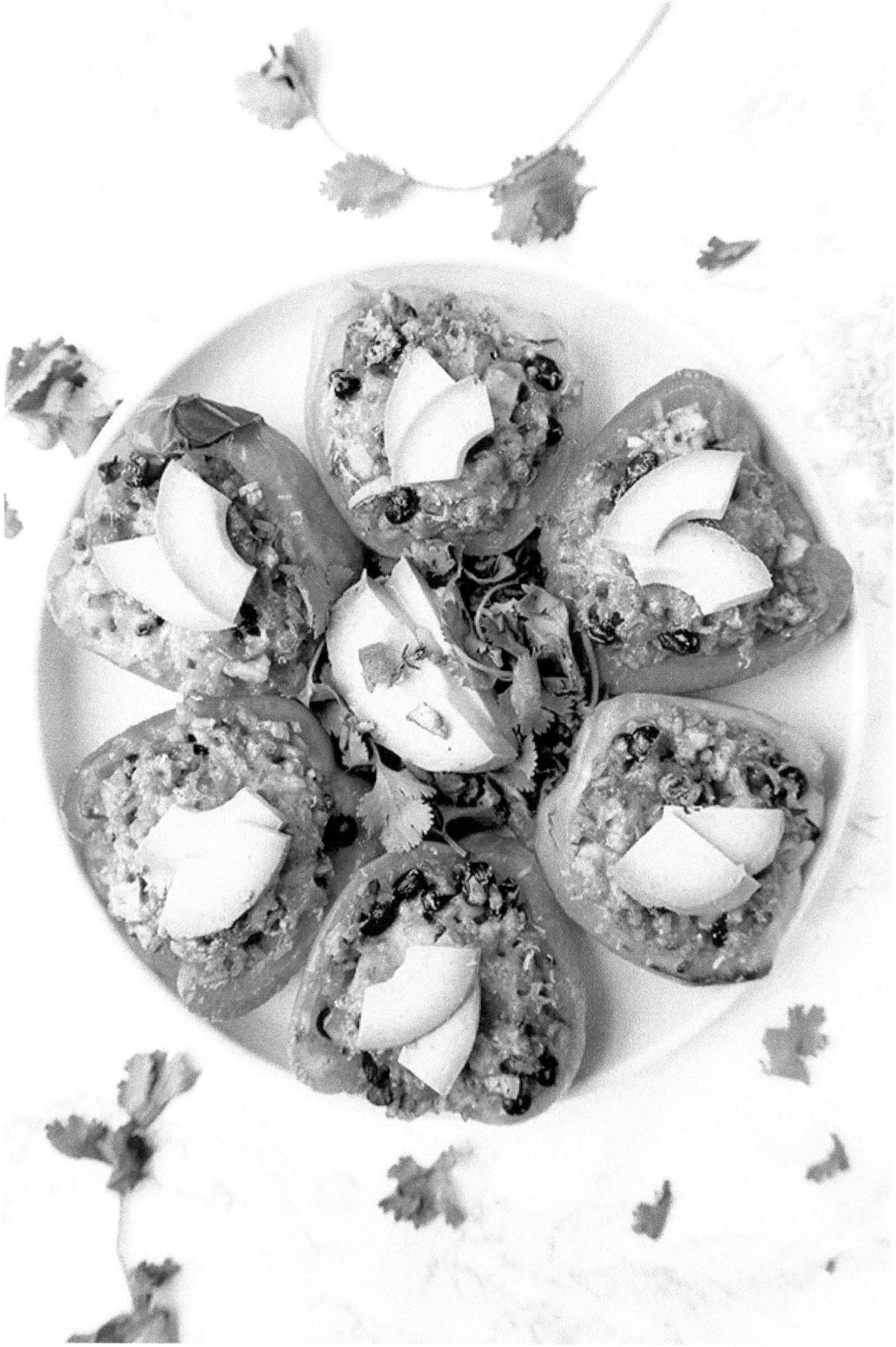

35 Kale Bake

(Ready in about 35 minutes | Serving 4 | Difficulty: Moderate)

Per serving: Kcal 384, Fat: 29.1g, Net Carbs: 5.9g, Protein: 25.1g

Ingredients

- Nonstick cooking spray
- 6 ounces kale, torn into pieces
- 4 eggs, whisked
- 1 cup Cheddar cheese, grated
- 1 cup Romano cheese
- 2 tbsp sour cream
- 1 garlic clove, minced
- Sea salt, to taste
- 1/2 tsp ground black pepper, or more to taste
- 1/2 tsp cayenne pepper

Instructions

Preheat the oven to 365 degrees F. Spray pan using cooking spray and mix everything in a bowl. Pour mixture into the prepared pan and bake for around 35 minutes.

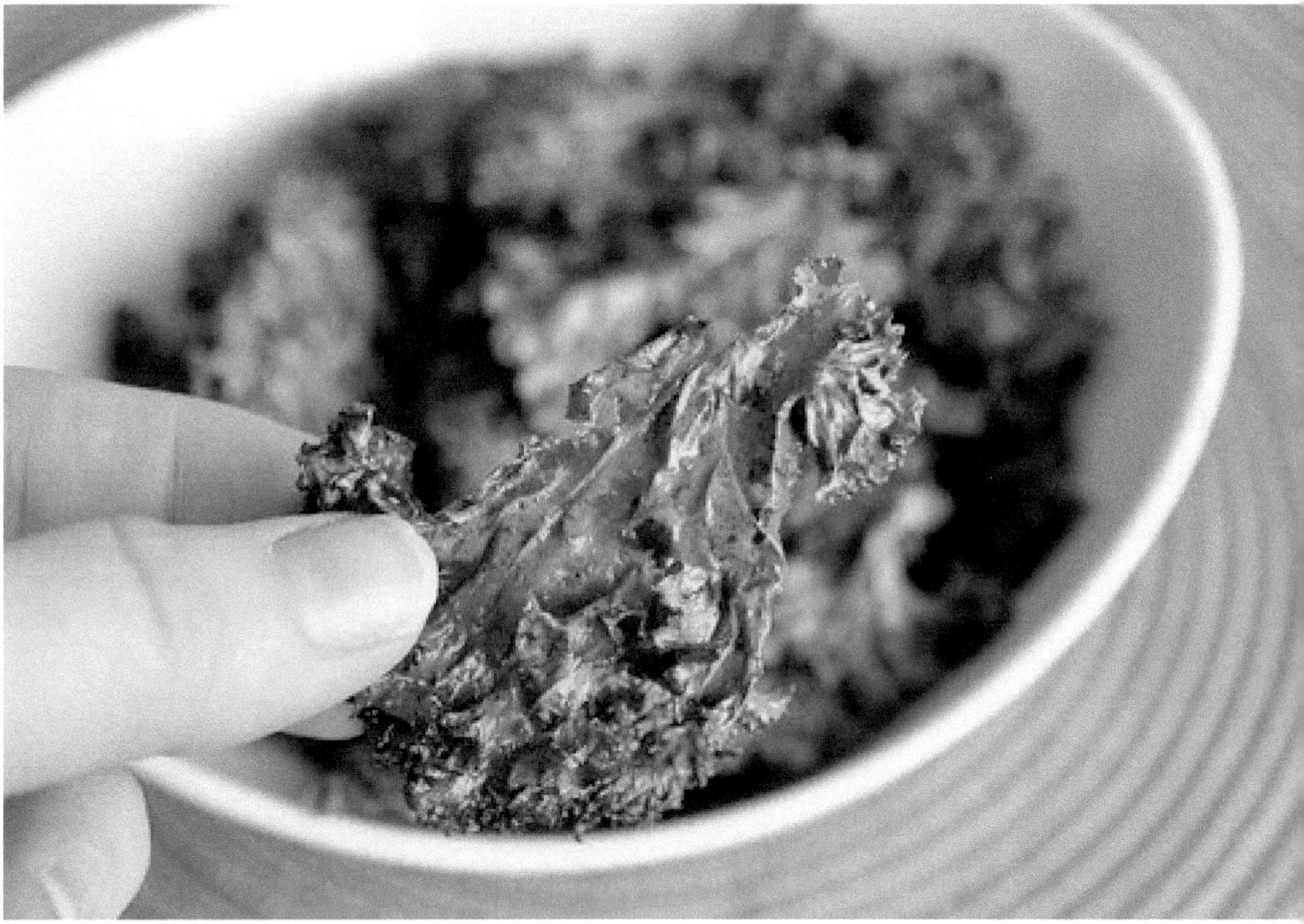

36 Cheese Meatballs

(Ready in about 25 minutes | Serving 8 | Difficulty: Easy)

Per serving: Kcal 389, Fat: 31.3g, Net Carbs: 1.6g, Protein: 23.8

Ingredients

- 1/2 pound ground pork
- 1 pound ground turkey
- 1 garlic clove, minced
- 4tbsp pork rinds, crushed
- 2 tbsp shallots, chopped
- 4 ounces mozzarella string cheese, cubed
- 1 ripe tomato, pureed
- Salt and ground black pepper, to taste

Instructions

Combine all the ingredients in a bowl except cheese. Shape eatable balls out of this mixture. Add cheese cube in every ball and line a baking sheet with parchment paper. Place balls on a sheet and bake for around 25 minutes at around 350 degrees F.

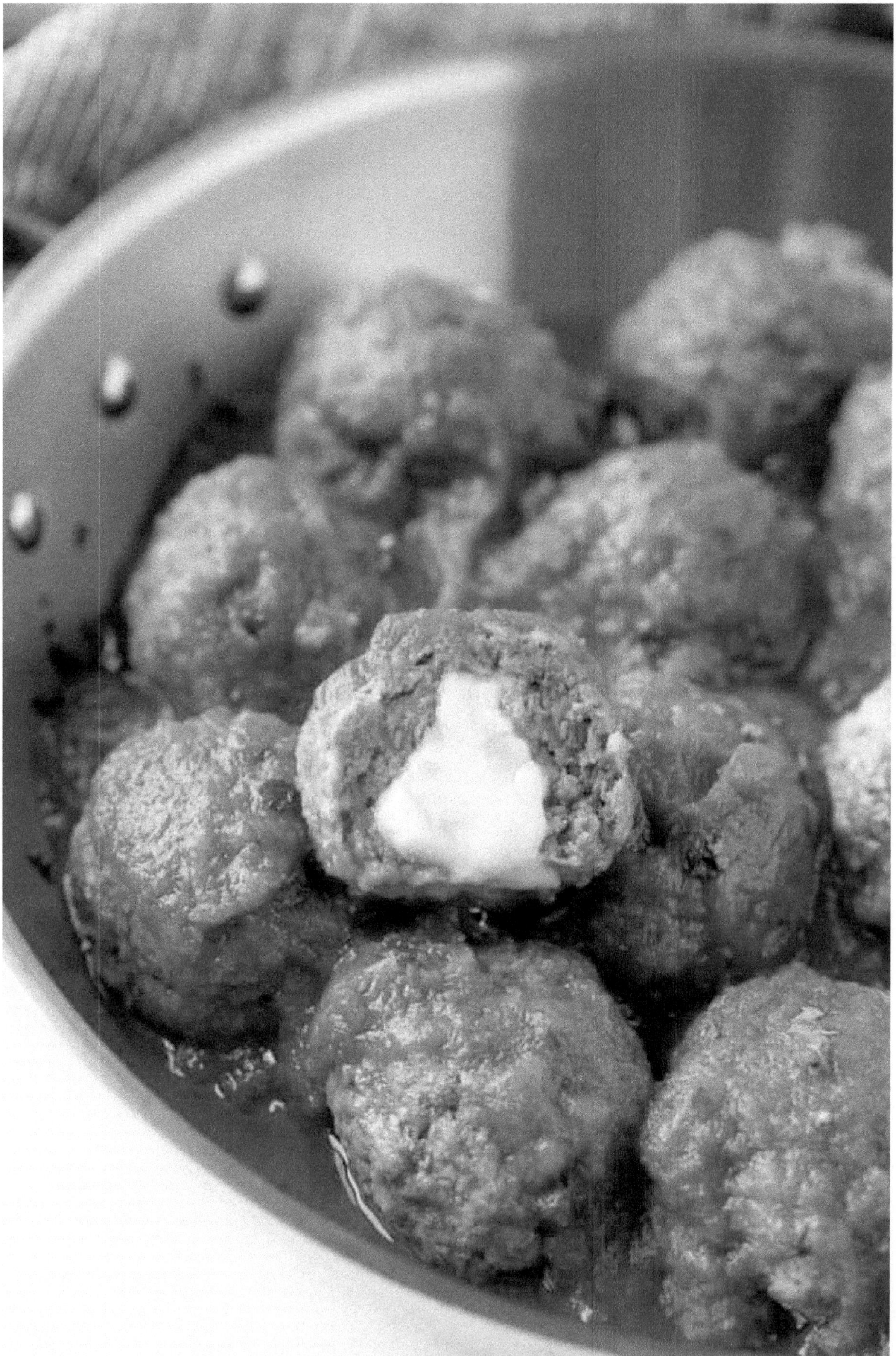

37 Italian Crisps

(Ready in about 10 minutes | Serving 4 | Difficulty: Easy)

Per serving: Kcal 134, Fat: 11.1g, Net Carbs: 0.4g, Protein: 4.9g

Ingredients

- 1 cup sharp Cheddar cheese, grated
- 1/4 tsp ground black pepper
- 1/2tsp cayenne pepper
- 1 tsp Italian seasoning

Instructions

Preheat the oven to 400 degrees F and line parchment paper on a baking sheet. Mix everything in a bowl and pour onto a sheet in for of heaps of the size of a tbsp. Bake for around 8 minutes.

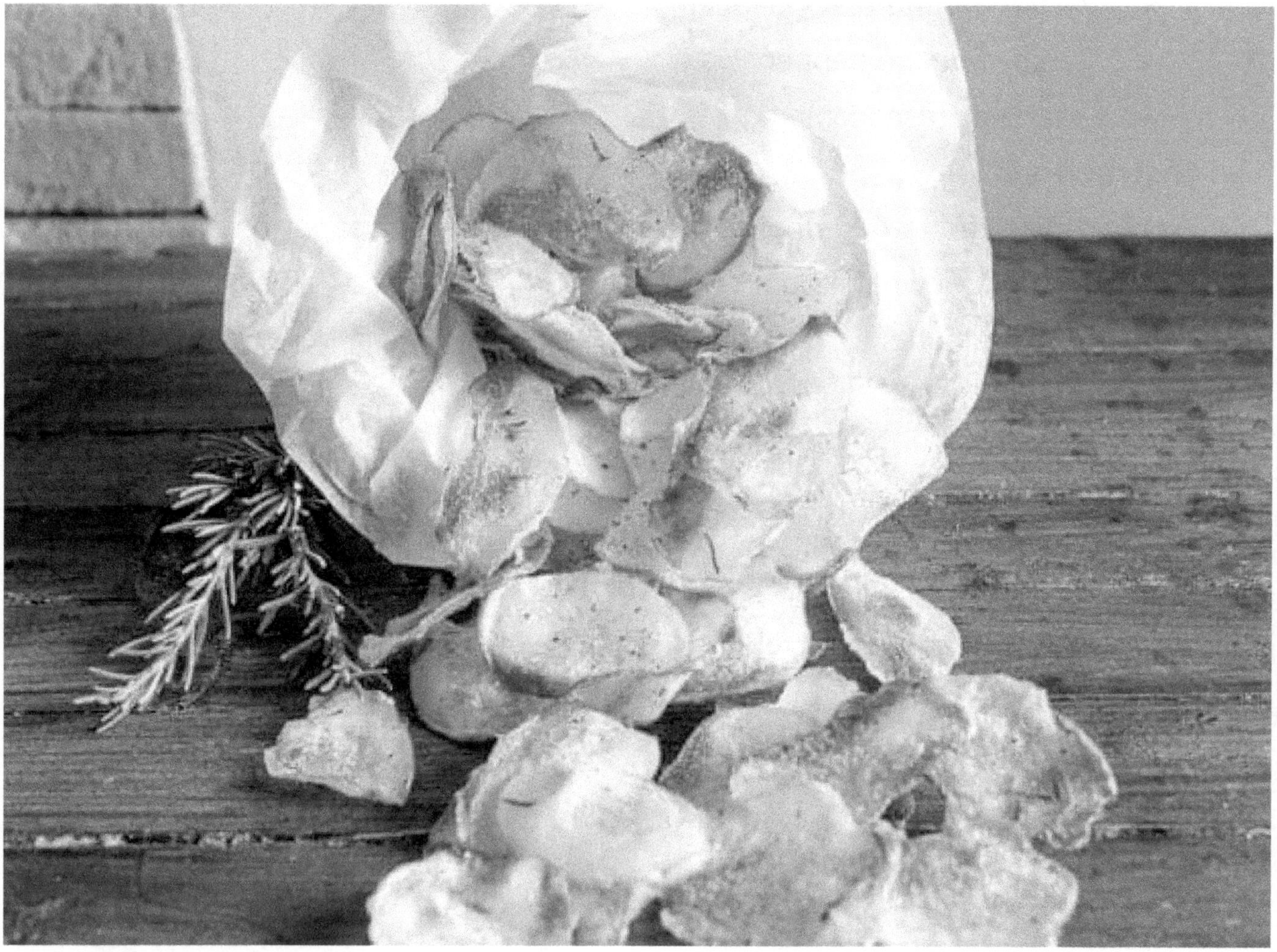

38 Spicy Meatballs

(Ready in about 15 minutes | Serving 3 | Difficulty: Easy)

Per serving: Kcal 458, Fat: 35.8g, Net Carbs: 4.3g, Protein: 28.2g

Ingredients

Sauce

- 3 ounces Asiago cheese, grated
- 1/4 cup mayonnaise
- 1 chili pepper, minced
- 1 tsp yellow mustard
- 1 tsp Italian parsley
- 1/2 tsp red pepper flakes, crushed
- 1/2 tsp sea salt
- 1/2 tsp ground black pepper

Meatballs

- 1/2 pound ground beef
- 1 egg
- 1 tbsp olive oil

Instructions

Add all the ingredients in the bowl except egg and beef and mix. Add egg and beef and combine thoroughly. Make meatballs out of the mixture. Warm oil in a pan placed on a moderate flame. Cook each side of meatballs for around 3 minutes.

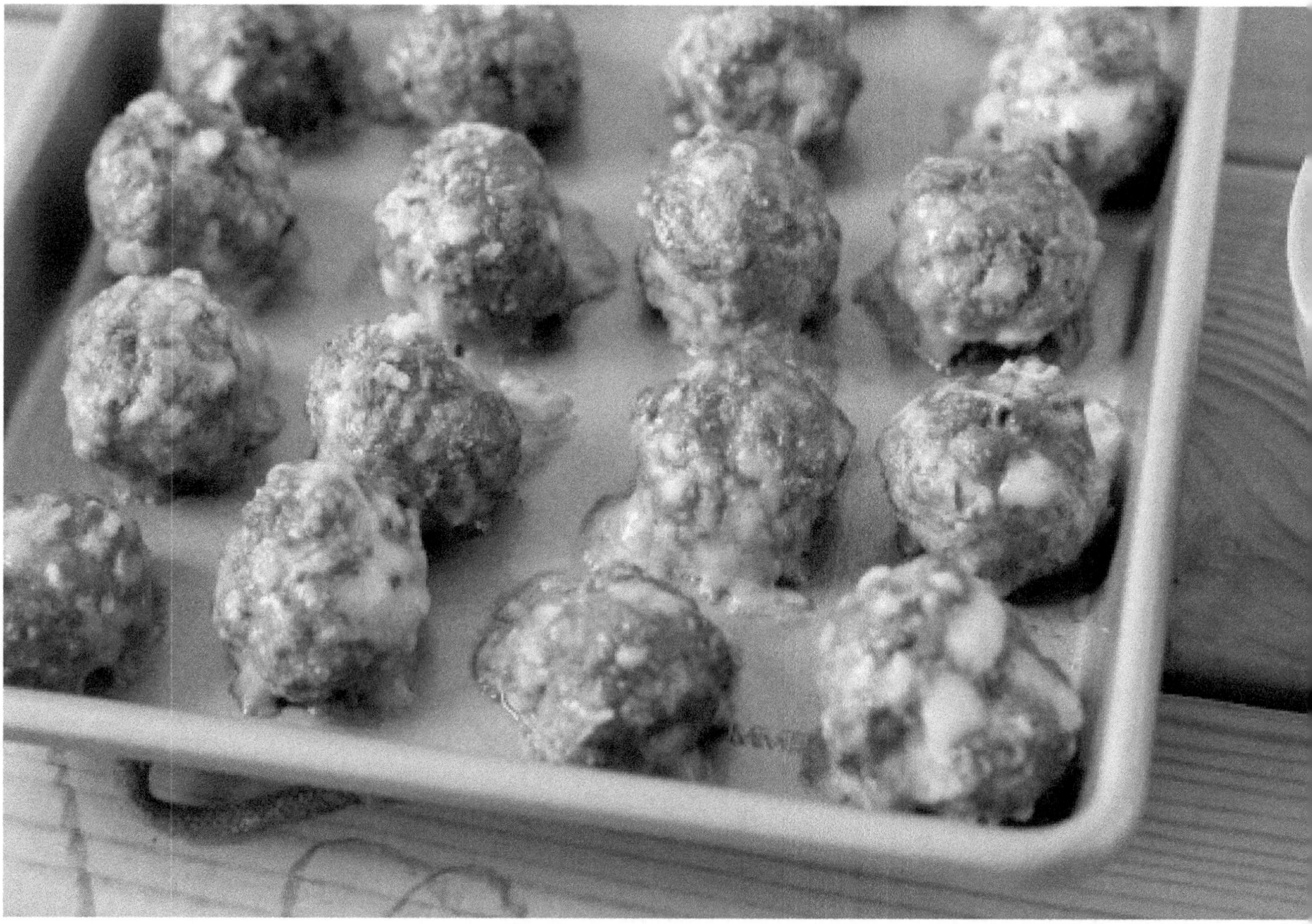

39 Cheese Stuffed Mushrooms

(Ready in about 25 minutes | Serving 5 | Difficulty: Easy)

Per serving: Kcal 148, Fat: 8.4g, Net Carbs: 4.8g, Protein: 14.1g

Ingredients

- 4 ounces ground beef
- 2 ounces ground pork
- Kosher salt and ground black pepper, to taste
- 1/4 cup goat cheese, crumbled
- 2 tbsp Romano cheese, grated
- 2 tbsp shallot, minced
- 1 garlic clove, minced
- 1 tsp dried basil
- 1/2 tsp dried oregano
- 1/2 tsp dried rosemary
- 20 button mushrooms, stems removed

Instructions

Add everything except mushrooms in a bowl and mix. Stuff this mixture inside mushrooms. Preheat the oven to 370 degrees F. Bake these mushrooms in a pan for around 18 minutes.

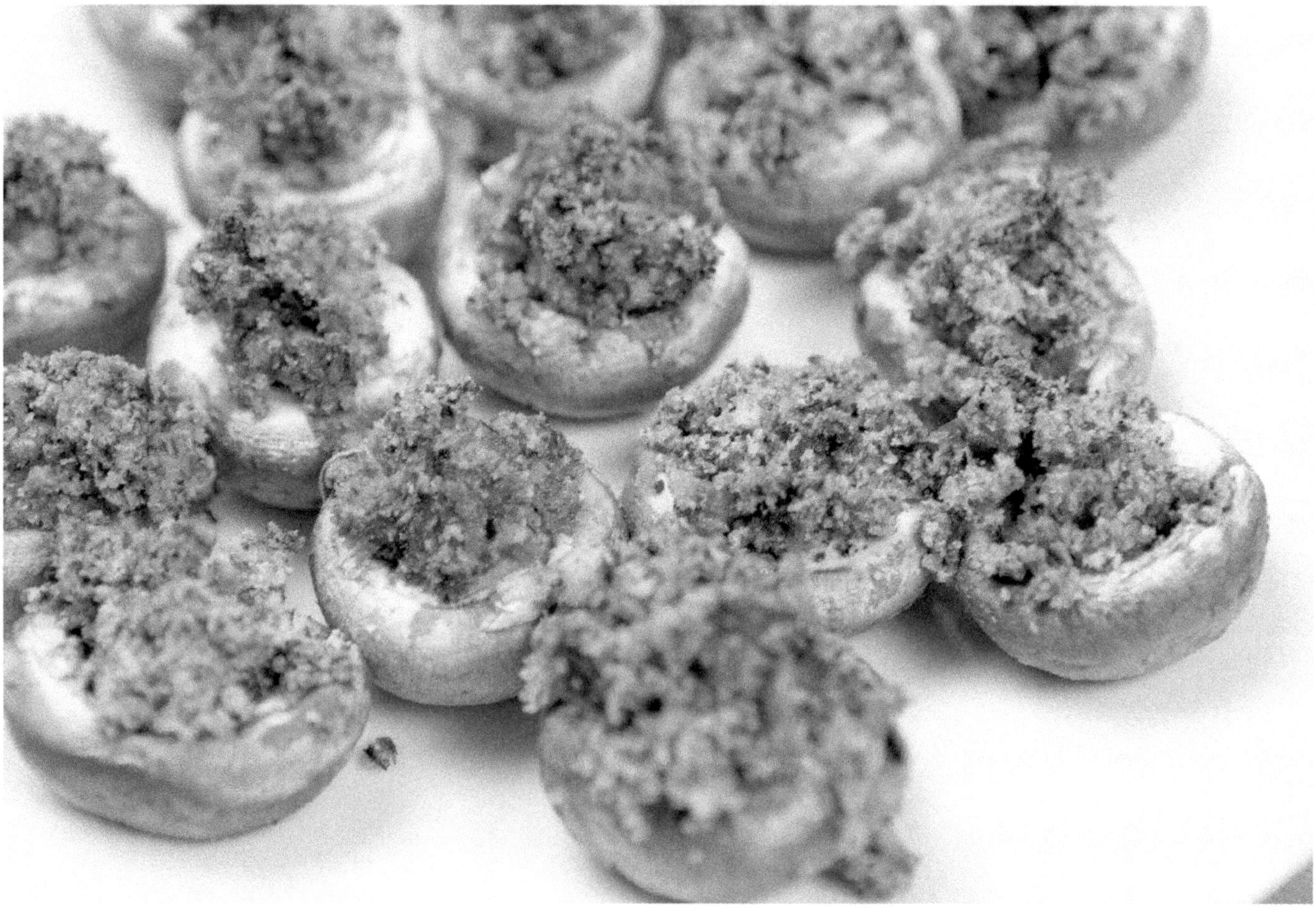

40 Beef with Herbs

(Ready in about 50 minutes | Serving 4 | Difficulty: Moderate)

Per serving: Kcal 421, Fat: 35.7g, Net Carbs: 5.9g, Protein: 19.7g

Ingredients

- 1 tbsp olive oil
- 1 pound rib eye, cut into strips
- 2 tbsp rice wine
- 1/4cup beef bone broth
- Sea salt and ground black pepper, to taste
- 2 tbsp fresh parsley, finely chopped
- 2 tbsp fresh chives, finely chopped
- 2chipotle peppers in adobo sauce, chopped
- 1 garlic clove, crushed
- 2 small-sized ripe tomatoes, pureed
- 1 yellow onion, peeled and chopped
- 1/2 tsp dry mustard
- 1 tsp dried basil
- 1 tsp dried marjoram

Instructions

Warm oil in a pan placed on a moderate flame. Sear beef in pan for around 6 minutes. Reduce flame and add the rest of the ingredients and cook for around 40 minutes. Take the beef out and shred and enjoy.

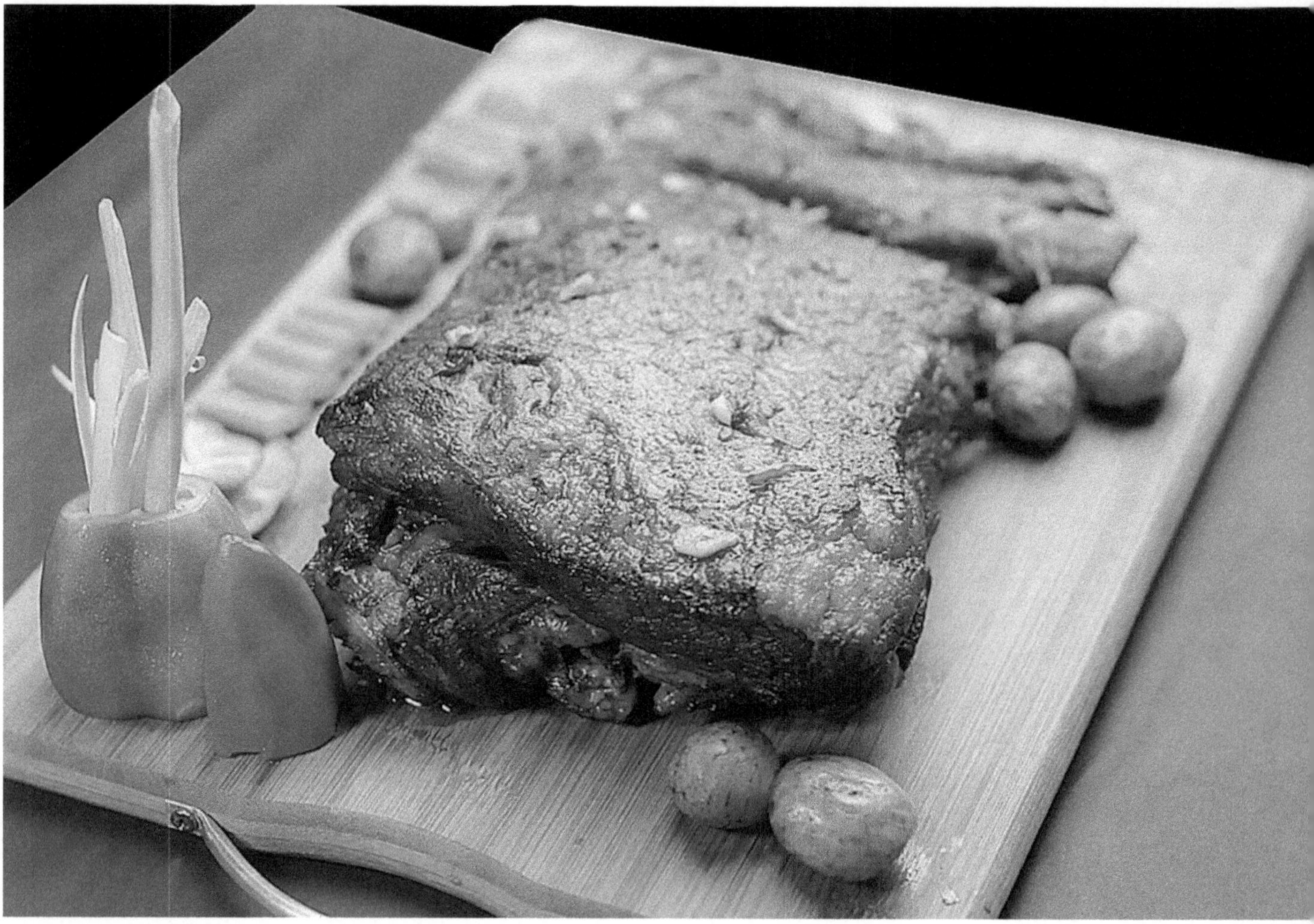

41 Chinese Beef Skillet

(Ready in about 15 minutes | Serving 3 | Difficulty: Easy)

Per serving: Kcal 179, Fat: 10.4g, Net Carbs: 5.8g, Protein: 16.5g

Ingredients

- 1 tbsp sesame oil
- 1/2 pound ground chuck
- 1 shallot, minced
- 1 garlic clove, minced
- 1 (1/2-inch) piece ginger root, peeled and grated
- 1 bell pepper, seeded and sliced
- 4 ounces brown mushrooms, sliced
- 1 tsp tamari soy sauce
- 1 tbsp rice wine
- 2 whole star anise
- Himalayan salt and ground black pepper, to taste

Instructions

Warm oil in a pan over moderate flame and cook chuck until it changed its color. Then cook veggies in drippings inside the pan. Add rest of ingredients and beef to pan. Reduce flame and simmer for around 3 minutes.

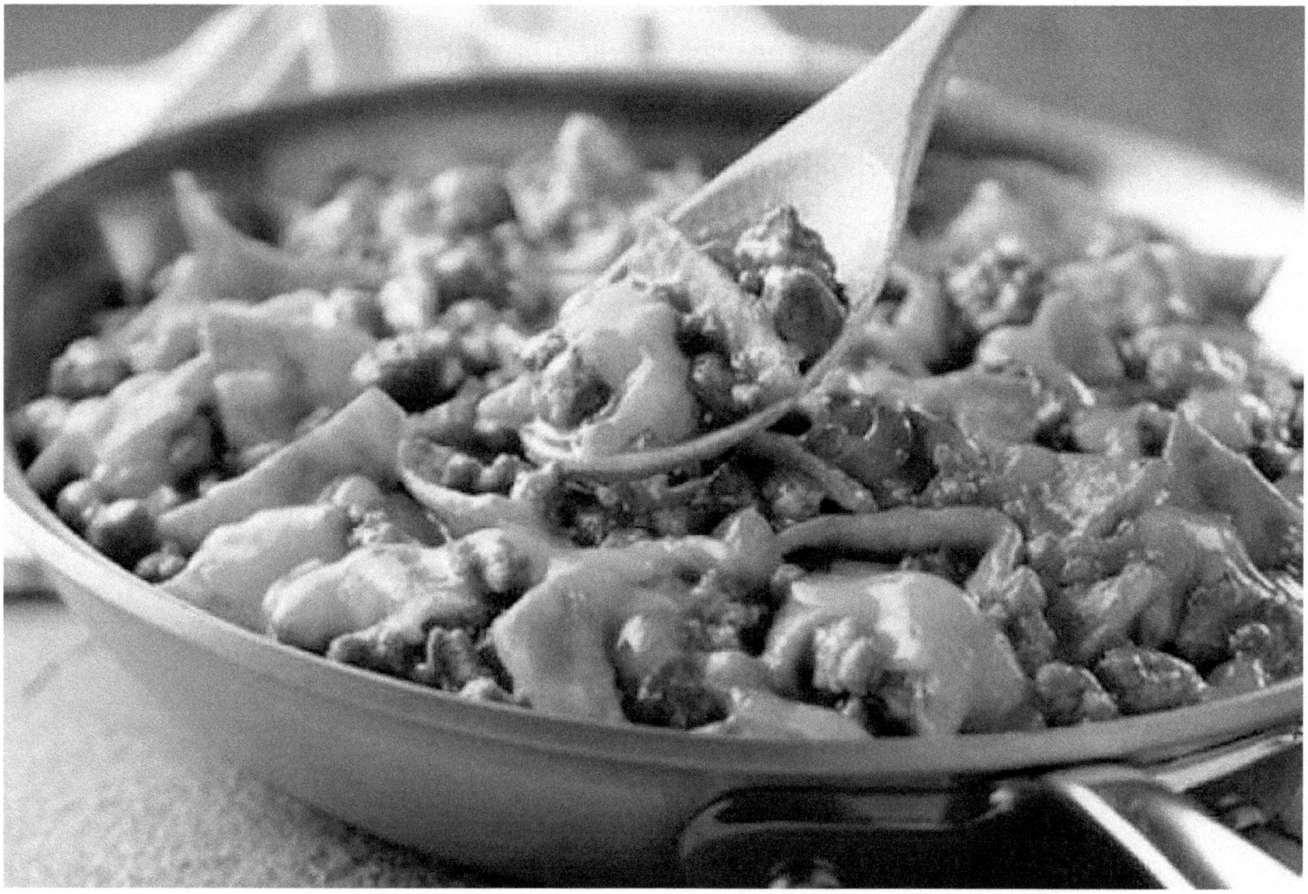

42 Beef Stroganoff

(Ready in about 1 hour | Serving 4 | Difficulty: Hard)

Per serving: Kcal 303, Fat: 17.2g, Net Carbs: 5.6g, Protein: 32.4g

Ingredients

- 2 tbsp lard, room temperature
- 1 pound beef stew meat, cut across the grain into strips
- 1/2 yellow onion, peeled and chopped
- 2 garlic cloves, minced
- 4ounces fresh mushrooms, sliced
- 1/2 tsp salt
- 1 tsp smoked paprika
- 1/4tsp black pepper
- 1/2 tsp dried basil
- 1/4 cup red cooking wine
- 4 cups vegetable broth
- 1 fresh tomato, pureed
- 2 celery stalks, chopped
- 1/2 cup sour cream

Instructions

Place stockpot over moderate flame and melt the lard in it. Cook meat until it turns brown. Add garlic and onion and cook for around 1 minute. Add mushrooms, and until they turn tender, cook. Add rest of ingredients except sour cream and seasonings and simmer for around 50 minutes, covered. Add sour cream after turning the heat off and mix.

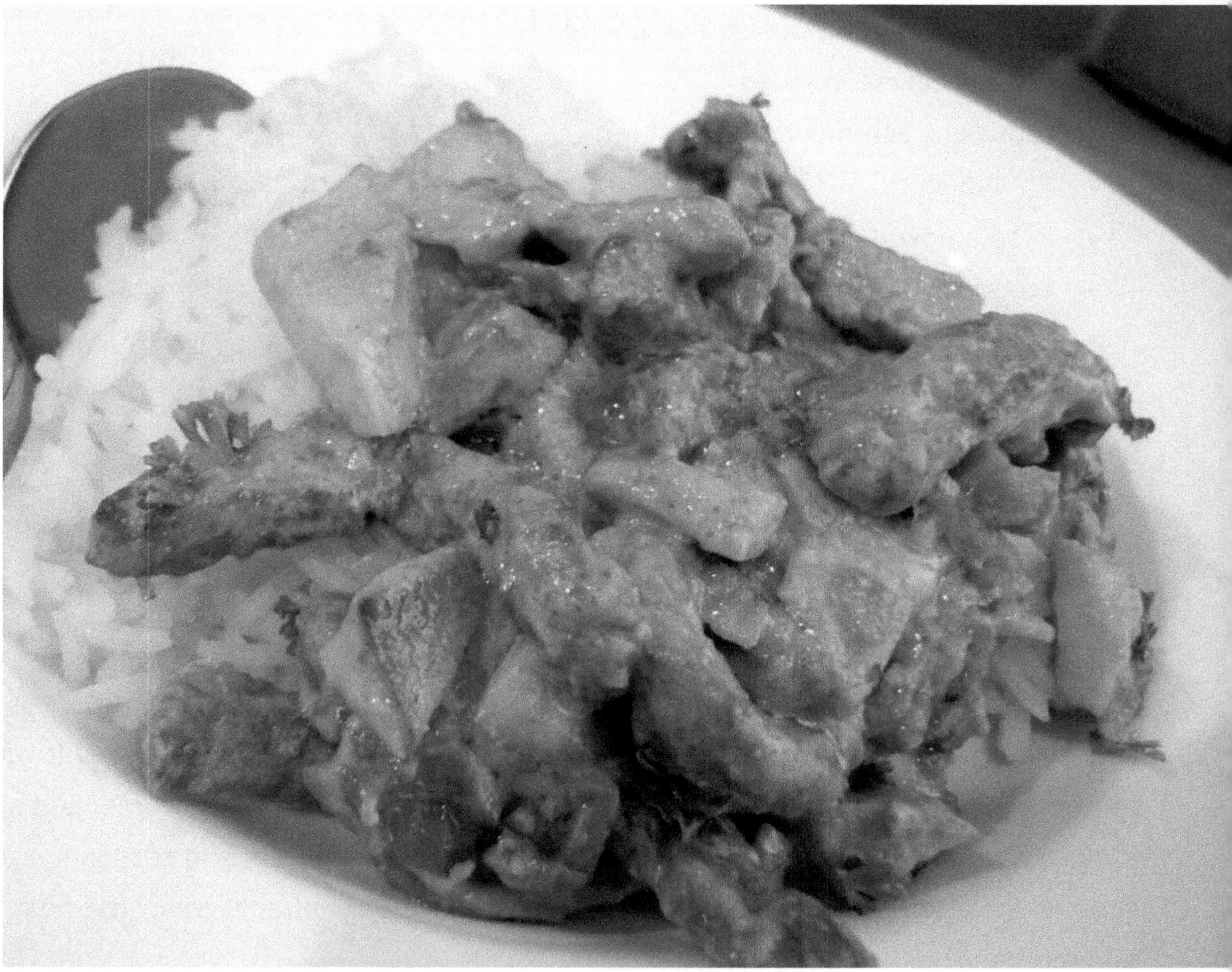

43 Chicken Zoodles

(Ready in about 19 minutes | Serving 4 | Difficulty: Easy)

Per serving: Kcal 411, Fat: 18.8g, Net Carbs: 11.7g, Protein: 45.7g

Ingredients

- 1/2 tsp of coconut butter
- 500 g of chicken fillets
- 1 medium onion diced
- 1 garlic minced
- Two zucchinis medium
- 400 g tomatoes crushed
- 100 g of raw cashews
- 7-10 chopped cherry tomatoes
- Salt, pepper, basil and oregano

Instructions

Warm pan over moderate flame. Cook butter and onions for around 1 minute. Make 2 cm pieces of chicken. Add garlic and chicken to the pan and sprinkle with seasonings. Cook for around 6 minutes. Spiralize zucchini in the meantime. Add tomatoes(crushed) and simmer for around 5 minutes. Roast cashews using another pan. Season with salt, paprika and turmeric. Add cherry tomatoes, zoodles and season using salt. Cook for another minute. Serve zoodles with fresh basil and cashews.

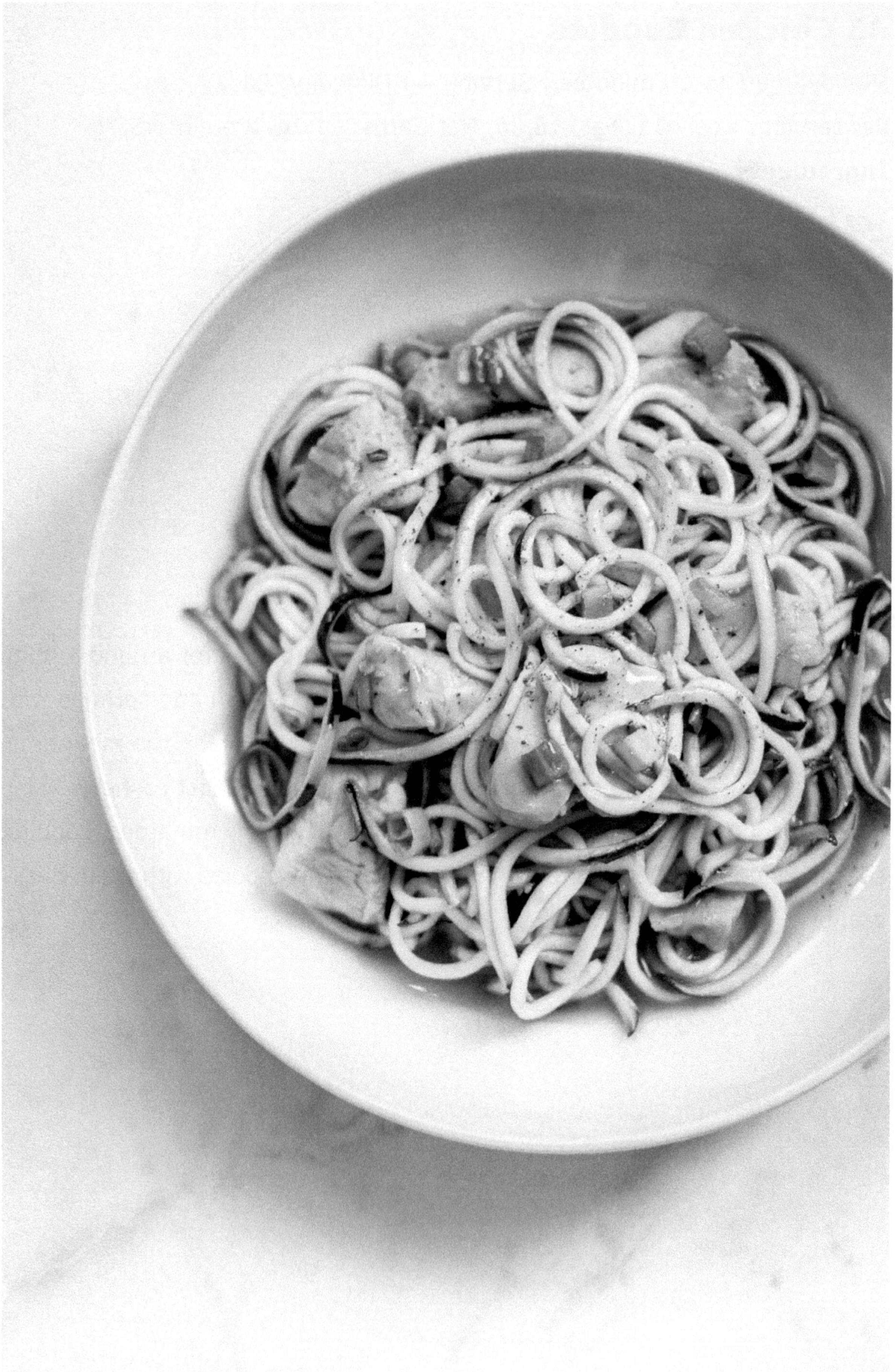

44 Creamy Tuscan Chicken

(Ready in about 25 minutes | Serving 6 | Difficulty: Easy)

Per serving: Kcal 368, Fat: 25g, Net Carbs: 7g, Protein: 30g

Ingredients

- 11/2 pounds of boneless skinless sliced chicken breasts
- 1 cup of heavy cream
- 1 cup chopped spinach
- 2 Tbsp of olive oil
- 1/2 cup of chicken broth
- 1 tsp of Italian seasoning
- 1 tsp of garlic powder
- 1/2 cup of parmesan cheese
- 1/2 cup of dried tomatoes

Instructions

Warm oil in a pan and cook each side of the chicken for around 5 minutes. Remove and place aside. Add everything except spinach and tomatoes to the pan and whisk over a moderate flame to form a thick mixture. Add tomatoes and spinach and simmer until spinach wilts. Add chicken and heat.

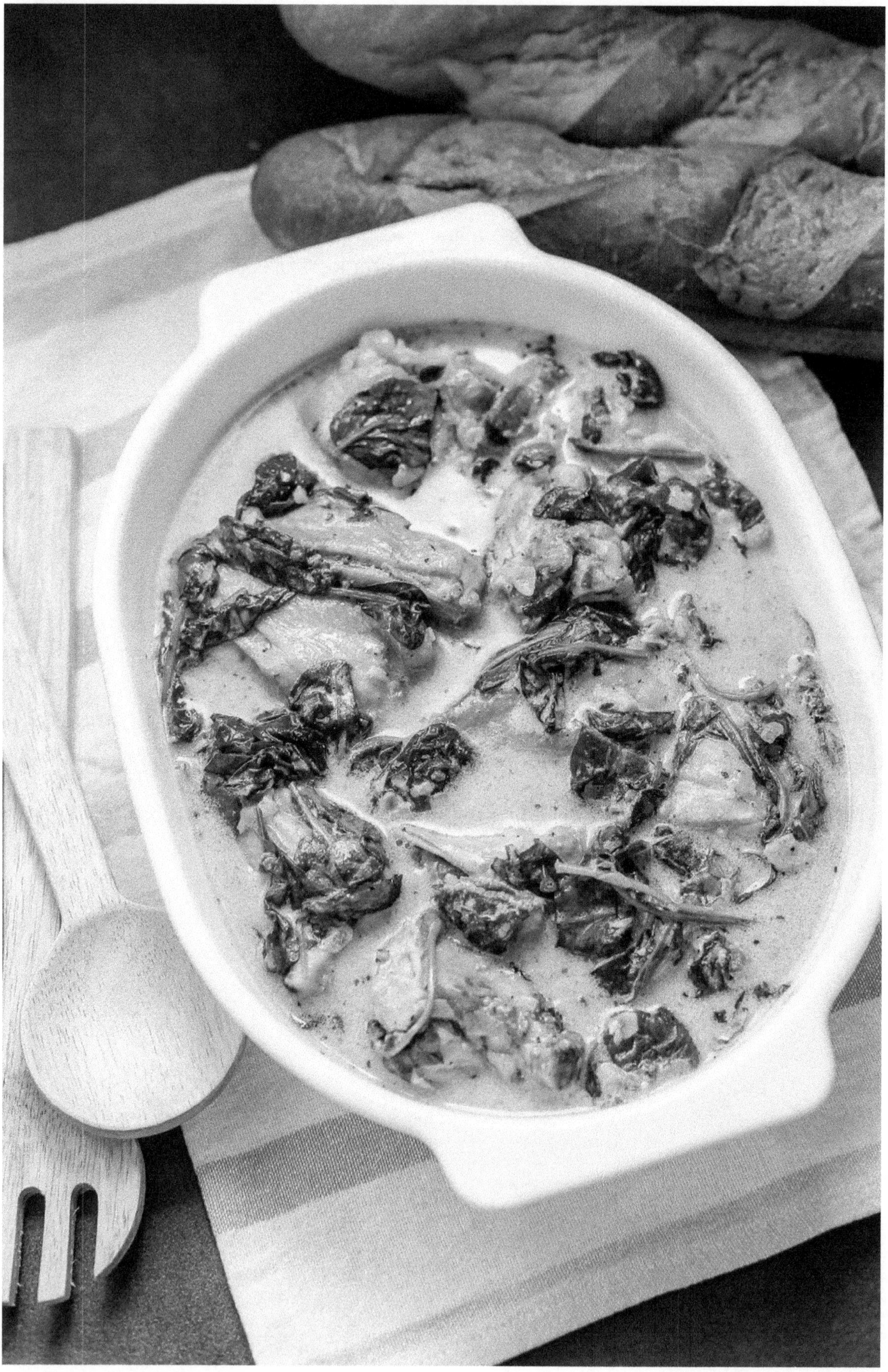

45 Turkey and peppers

(Ready in about 20 minutes | Serving 4 | Difficulty: Easy)

Per serving: Kcal 230, Fat: 8g, Net Carbs: 11g, Protein: 30g

Ingredients

- 1/2 large sliced sweet onion
- 1 pound cut into steaks turkey tenderloin
- 1 diced into strips yellow bell pepper
- 2 tbsp divided olive oil extra-virgin
- 1 diced into strips red bell pepper
- 1 tsp divided salt
- 1/2tsp of Italian seasoning
- 2 tsp of red wine vinegar
- 1/4tsp of ground black pepper
- 1 14-ounce can of crushed tomatoes

Instructions

Sprinkle turkey with half tsp salt. Warm 1 tbsp oil in a pan and cook half of the turkey for around 3 minutes. Transfer to a plate and add remaining oil to the pan. Repeat with the rest of the turkey. Add veggies and half tsp salt to the pan and cook for around 7 minutes. Sprinkle with seasoning plus pepper and cook on a moderate flame for around 30 seconds. Add vinegar and cook for another 20 seconds. Add turkey to the pan and simmer for around 2 minutes. Top with basil and parsley.

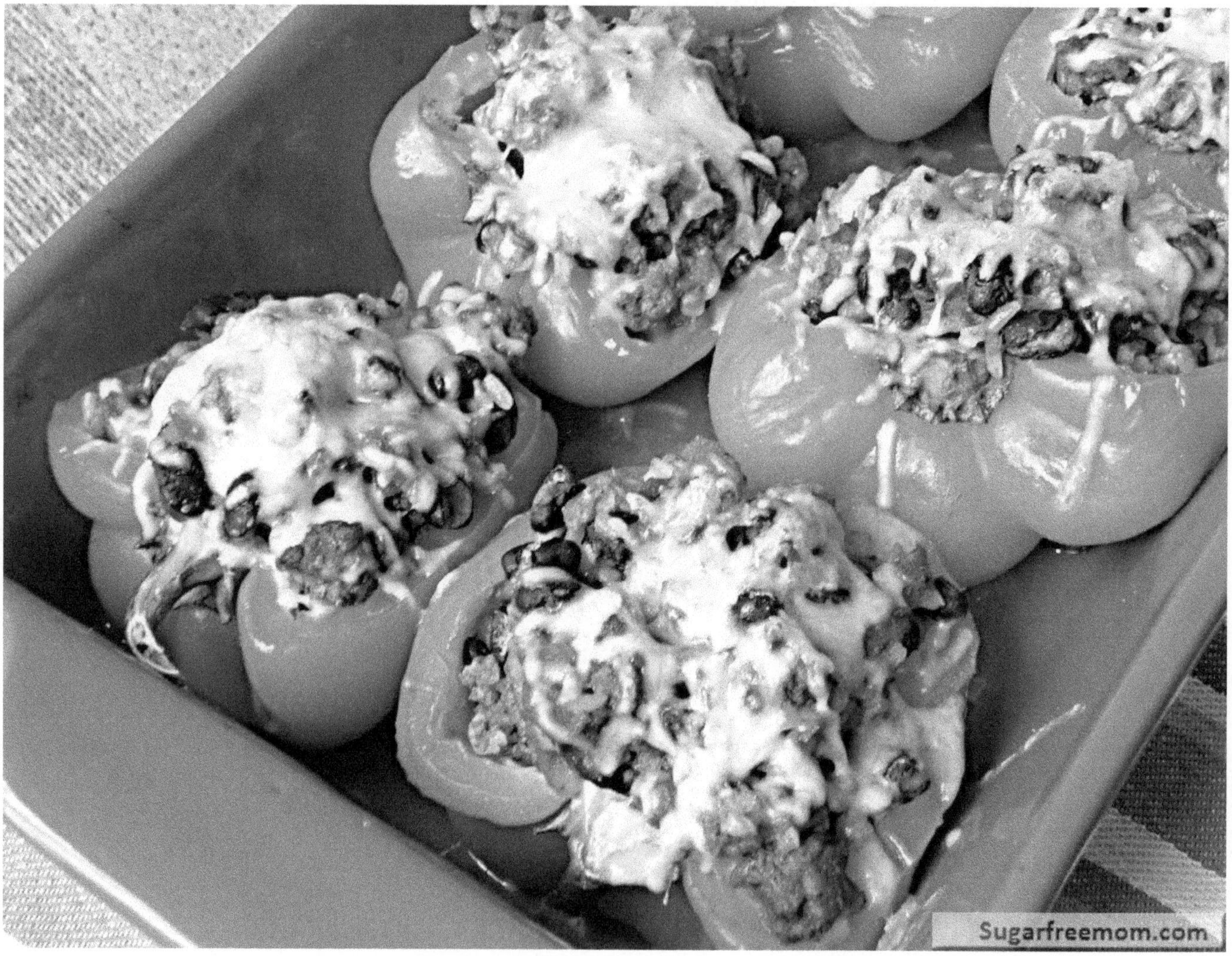
Sugarfreemom.com

46 Butter Chicken

(Ready in about 30 minutes | Serving 6 | Difficulty: Easy)

Per serving: Kcal 293, Fat: 17g, Net Carbs: 9g, Protein: 29g

Ingredients

- 1.5 lbs cubed chicken breast
- 4 oz plain Greek yogurt whole milk
- 3 tsp grated fresh ginger
- 2 tbsp of garam masala
- 3 tsp garlic minced
- 1 tbsp of coconut oil

Sauce

- 2 tbsp of butter
- 2 tsp grated fresh ginger
- 1/2 cup of heavy cream
- 2 tsp garlic minced
- 14.5 oz can tomatoes crushed
- 1 onion
- 1 tbsp coriander ground
- 2 tsp of cumin
- 1/2tbsp of garam masala
- 1 tsp of chili powder
- Salt

Instructions

Dice chicken into pieces of 2 inch and mix with garam masala, 1 tsp each of garlic and ginger in a bowl. Add yogurt and mix. Place in the fridge for around 30 minutes. Add tomatoes, garlic, ginger, spices and onion in a blender and blend to make a smooth mixture. Place aside. Warm 1 tbsp oil in a pan and add marinade and chicken. Cook each side for around 4 minutes. Add sauce and cook for 6 more minutes. Add ghee and heavy cream and cook for an additional minute. Top using cilantro.

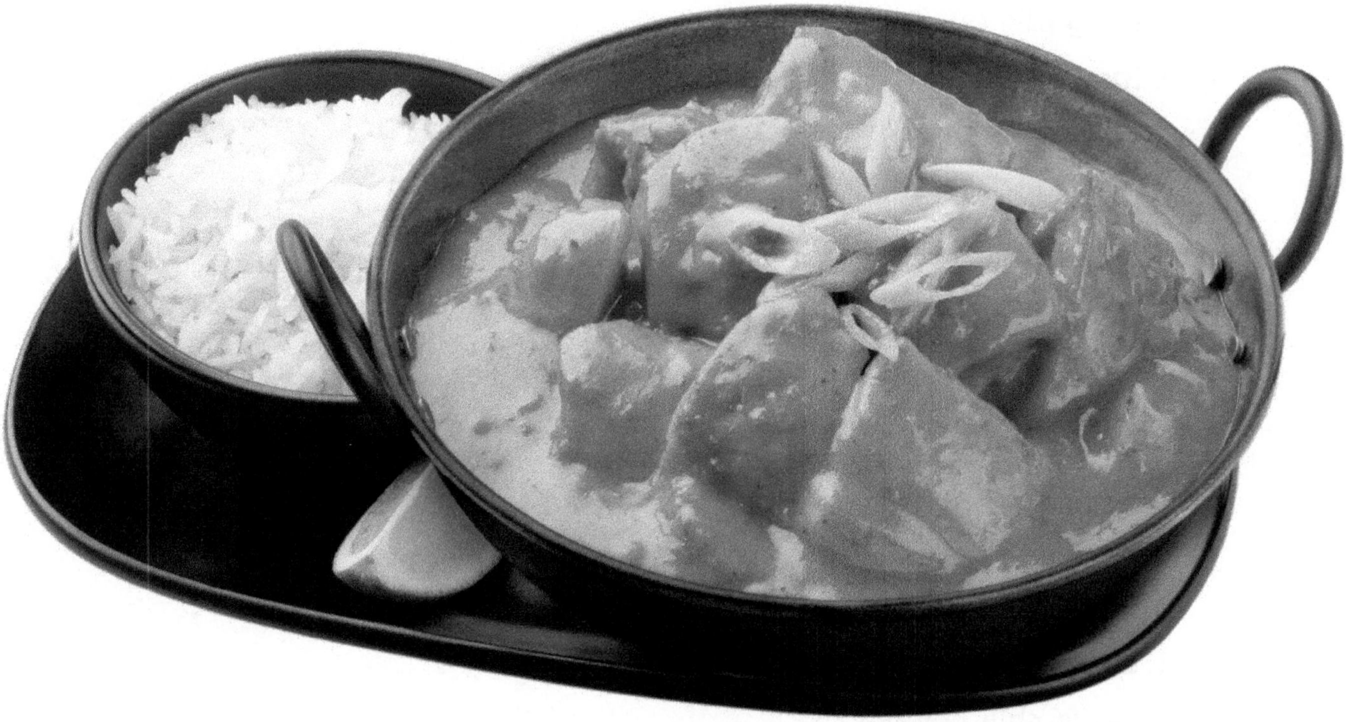

47 Asparagus Chicken

(Ready in about 30 minutes | Serving 3 | Difficulty: Easy)

Per serving: Kcal 572, Fat: 31g, Net Carbs: 10g, Protein: 62g

Ingredients

- 3 Breasts Chicken
- 12 Stalks removed Asparagus
- 1 cup of mozzarella shredded
- 1 tsp of Garlic paste
- 1/2 cup of Cream Cheese
- 1 tsp of Olive Oil
- 1 tbsp of Butter
- 3/4 cup of Marinara Sauce
- Pepper and salt

Instructions

Slice chicken without cutting from the center. Cut stalks from asparagus. Rub garlic paste, salt and pepper over chicken and spread with cream cheese. Place 4 asparagus stalks in the center and fold the breasts. Preheat the oven to 400 degrees F and cook each side for around 7 minutes. Top with marinara sauce and mozzarella. Broil for around 5 minutes.

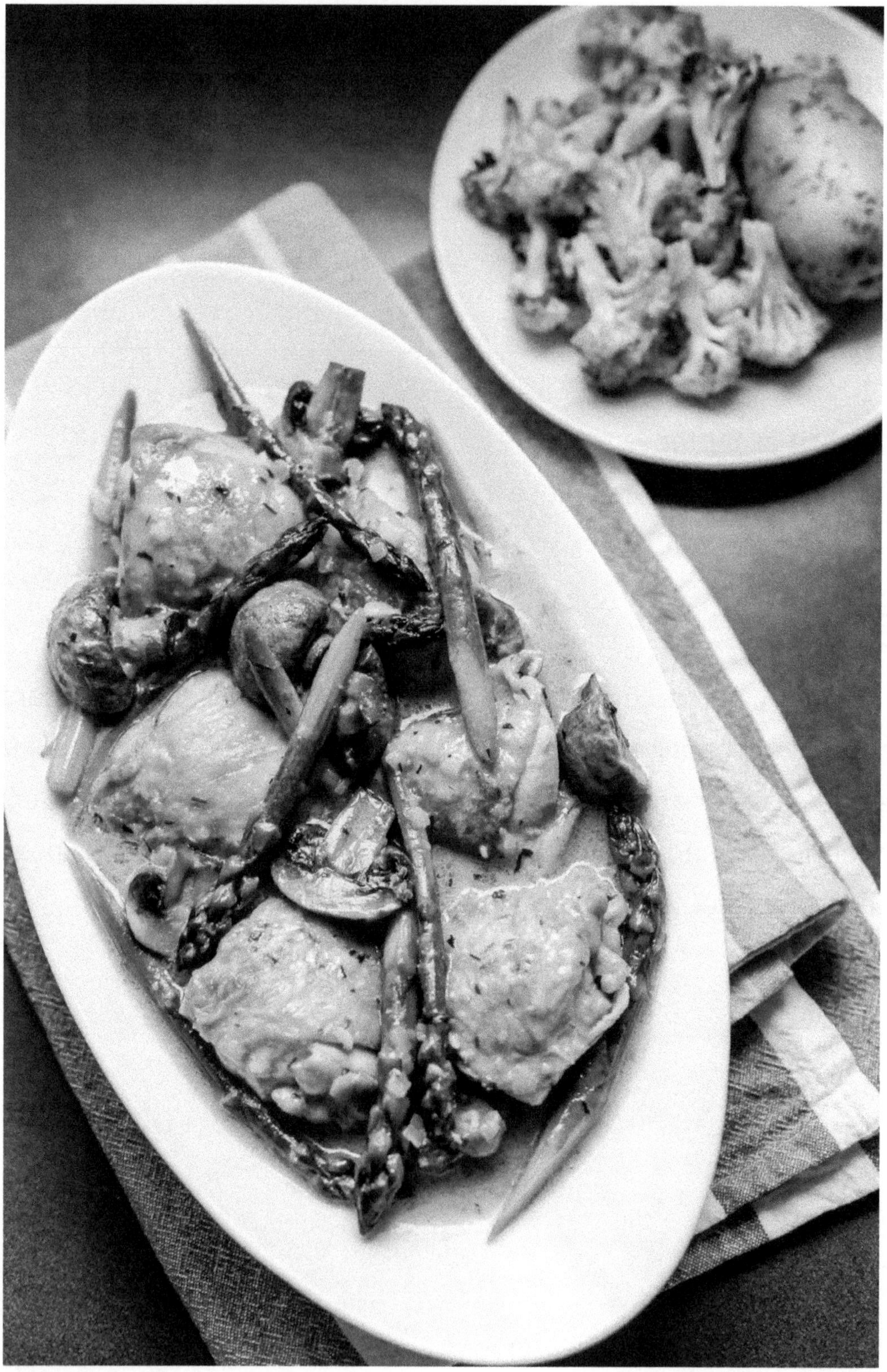

48 Chicken Chili

(Ready in about 30 minutes | Serving 6 | Difficulty: Easy)

Per serving: Kcal 201, Fat: 11g, Net Carbs: 7g, Protein: 18g

Ingredients

- 4 shredded chicken breasts
- 2 cups of Chicken broth
- 1 tbsp of Butter
- 1/2 chopped onion
- 10 oz canned diced tomatoes, undrained
- 4 oz of Cream cheese
- 2 oz of tomato paste
- 1 tbsp of Cumin
- 1 tbsp of Chili powder
- 1/2 tbsp of Garlic powder
- Pepper and salt

Instructions

Boil chicken in broth for around 12 minutes. Take out and shred. Melt butter in a pot over moderate flame and cook the onion for around 2 minutes. Add chicken and rest of the ingredients except cream cheese in pot and stir. Boil and reduce the flame to simmer for around 10 minutes. Cut cream into chunks of 1 inch. Add to pot and stir until mixed. Season using pepper and salt.

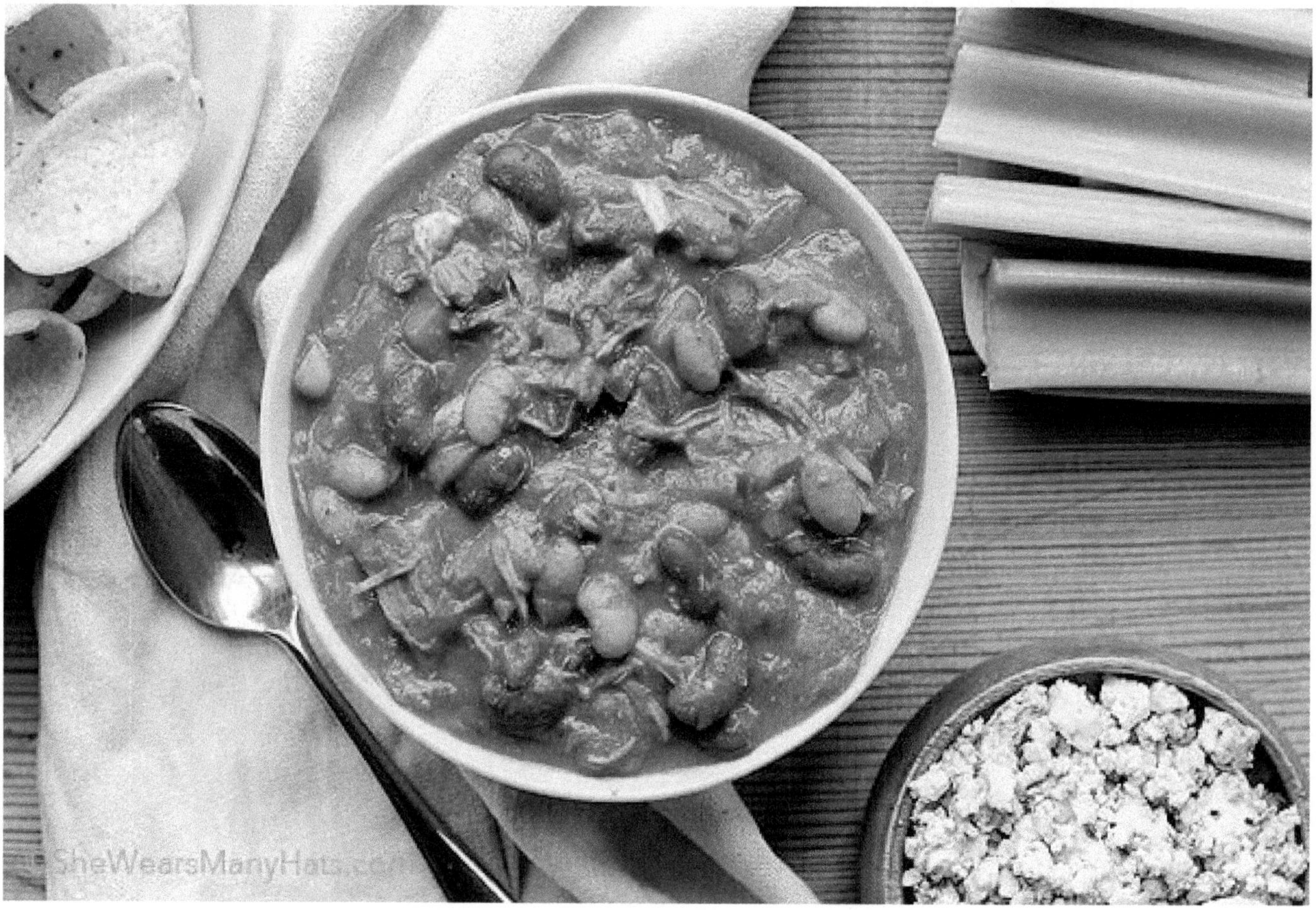

49 Taco Avocados

(Ready in about 20 minutes | Serving 6 | Difficulty: Easy)

Per serving: Kcal 401, Fat: 28g, Net Carbs: 5g, Protein: 26g

Ingredients

- 1 pound beef ground
- 1/2 tsp of Salt
- 1 tbsp of Chili Powder
- 1/2 tsp of Dried Oregano
- 3/4 tsp of Cumin
- 1/4 tsp of Garlic Powder
- 4 ounces of tomato sauce
- 1/4 tsp of Onion Powder
- 3 halved avocados
- 1 cup shredded cheddar cheese
- 1/4 cup sliced cherry tomatoes
- 1/4 cup shredded lettuce

Instructions

Add beef to a pan and cook until it turns brown. Remove grease and mix tomato sauce and seasonings. Cook for around 4 minutes and take the pit out of avocados. Load taco meat in crater and top with tomatoes, cheese, sour cream, cilantro and lettuce.

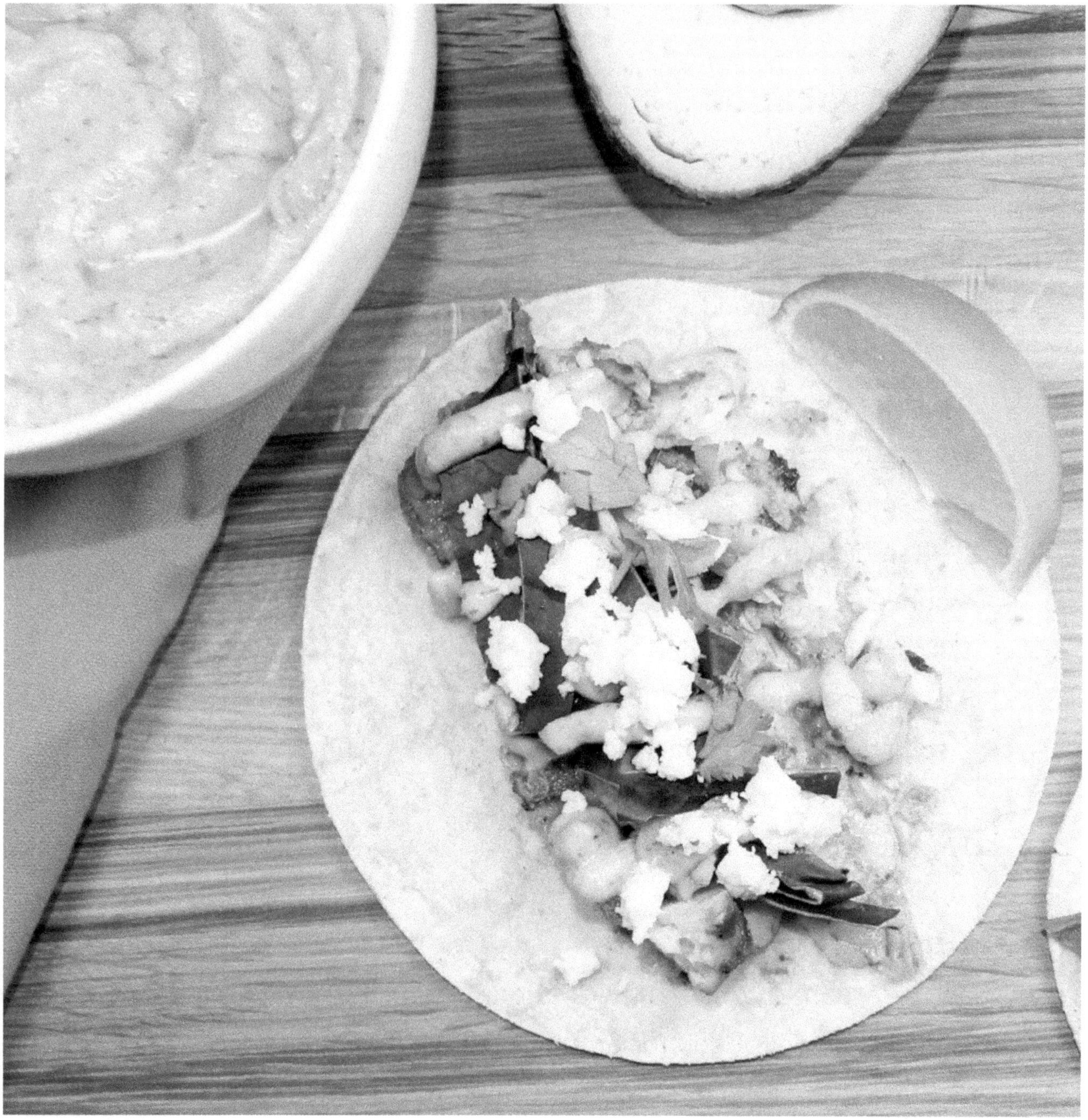

50 Broccoli Beef Bowls

(Ready in about 30 minutes | Serving 4 | Difficulty: Easy)

Per serving: Kcal 388, Fat: 29g, Net Carbs: 14g, Protein: 30g

Ingredients

Beef

- 1 pound grass-fed beef ground
- 1 tsp of granulated garlic
- 1 tsp of fine salt
- 1 tbsp of cooking fat
- 1 tbsp of coconut aminos

Broccoli

- 4 diced into florets broccoli crowns
- 1/2 tsp of fine salt
- 1 tbsp of avocado oil

Sunshine Sauce

- 1 tbsp of cooking fat
- 1/2 of fine salt
- 2 tbsp seed sunflower butter
- 2 tsp of coconut aminos
- 1 tsp of ground ginger
- one lemon, juiced
- 1 minced green onion
- 1/4 cup of bone broth

To assemble

- 4 cups of baby spinach

Instructions

Preheat oven to around 400 degrees F. Mix salt and fat with broccoli on pan and massage fat into florets. Cook for around 20 minutes. Crumble beef in a pan and add garlic and salt. Stir and add coconut aminos and turn flame to high. Cook until beef turns crispy and brown. Place a pot on moderate flame and melt fat in it. Add seed butter and sunflower and stir to make a smooth mixture. Add rest of ingredients except lemon juice and stir. Take off the heat and mix lemon juice. Add baby spinach to 4 bowls and divide beef equally. Add broccoli florets and top with sauce.

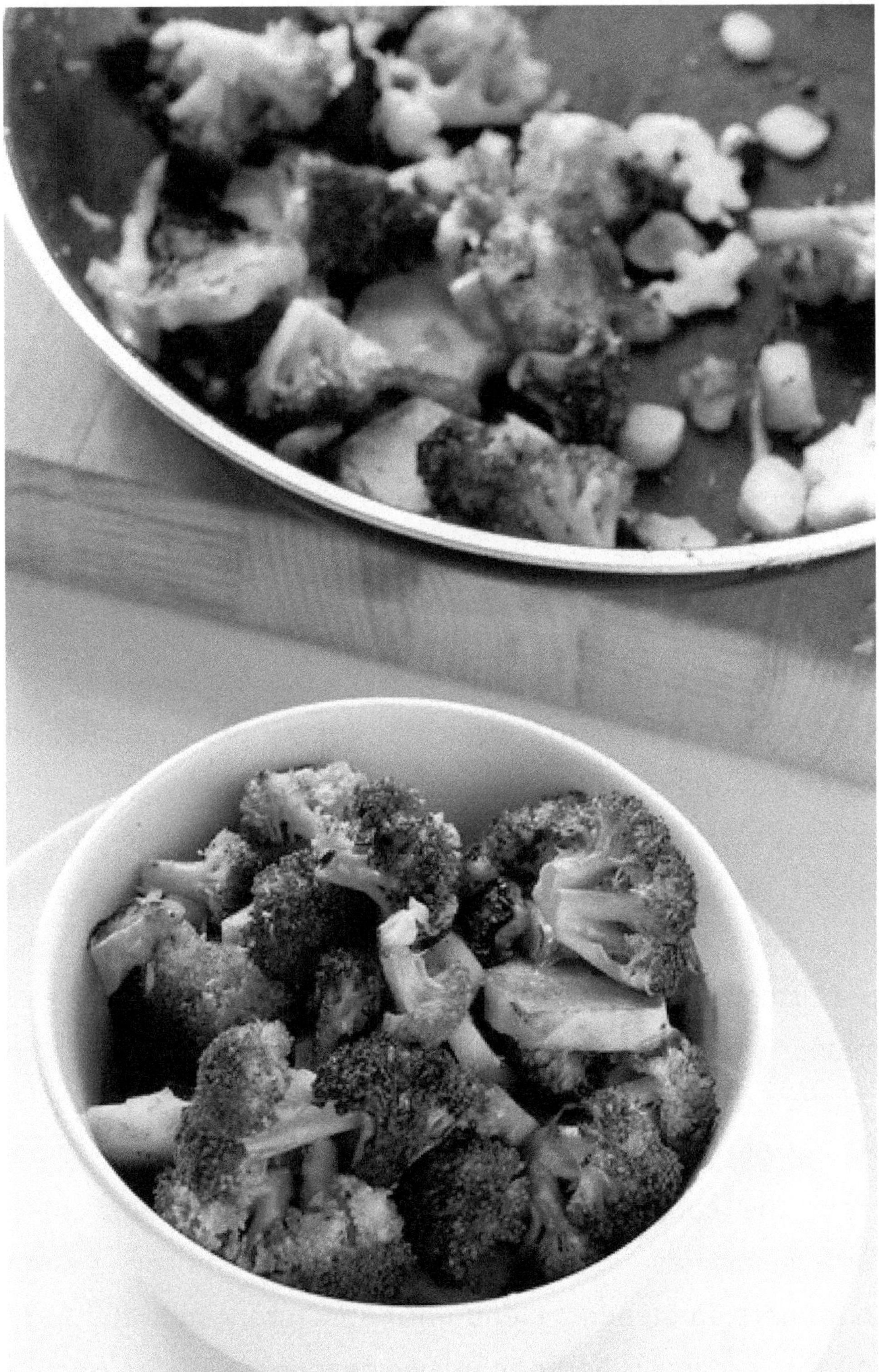

51 Cauliflower-Bacon Cheese Mash

(Ready in about 15 minutes | Serving 4 | Difficulty: Easy)

Per serving: Kcal 399, Fat: 32.2g, Sodium 877.8mg, Protein: 18.8g

Ingredients

- 1 cauliflower, large head, diced into florets
- ½ lb. bacon, diced
- 1 cup of Parmesan cheese, shredded
- 2 tbsp. medium-chain triglyceride oil
- 4 tbsp. unsalted butter
- Sea salt to taste
- ½ tbsp. apple cider vinegar

Instruction

- Cook the bacon in a big skillet over the medium-high flame, sometimes flipping, for five to ten minutes or evenly browned. Reserve the grease in the skillet and drain on the paper towels.
- In a pressure cooker, place the cauliflower in a metal or silicone steamer basket. Fill the container with 1 cup of water. Cover the lid and lock it. Set the timer for four minutes and select the Steam function. Allow for a ten to a fifteen-minute build-up of pressure.
- Pressure can be released slowly and cautiously using the quick-release system according to the manufacturer's directions, which should take around five minutes. Remove the lid by unlocking it.
- Drain the cauliflower and put it in a big mixing bowl. Combine the Parmesan cheese, butter, MCT oil, vinegar, and salt in a mixing bowl. Using an immersion blender, blend until absolutely smooth. Add the sliced bacon and mix properly. Add one or two teaspoons of the bacon grease that has been put aside.

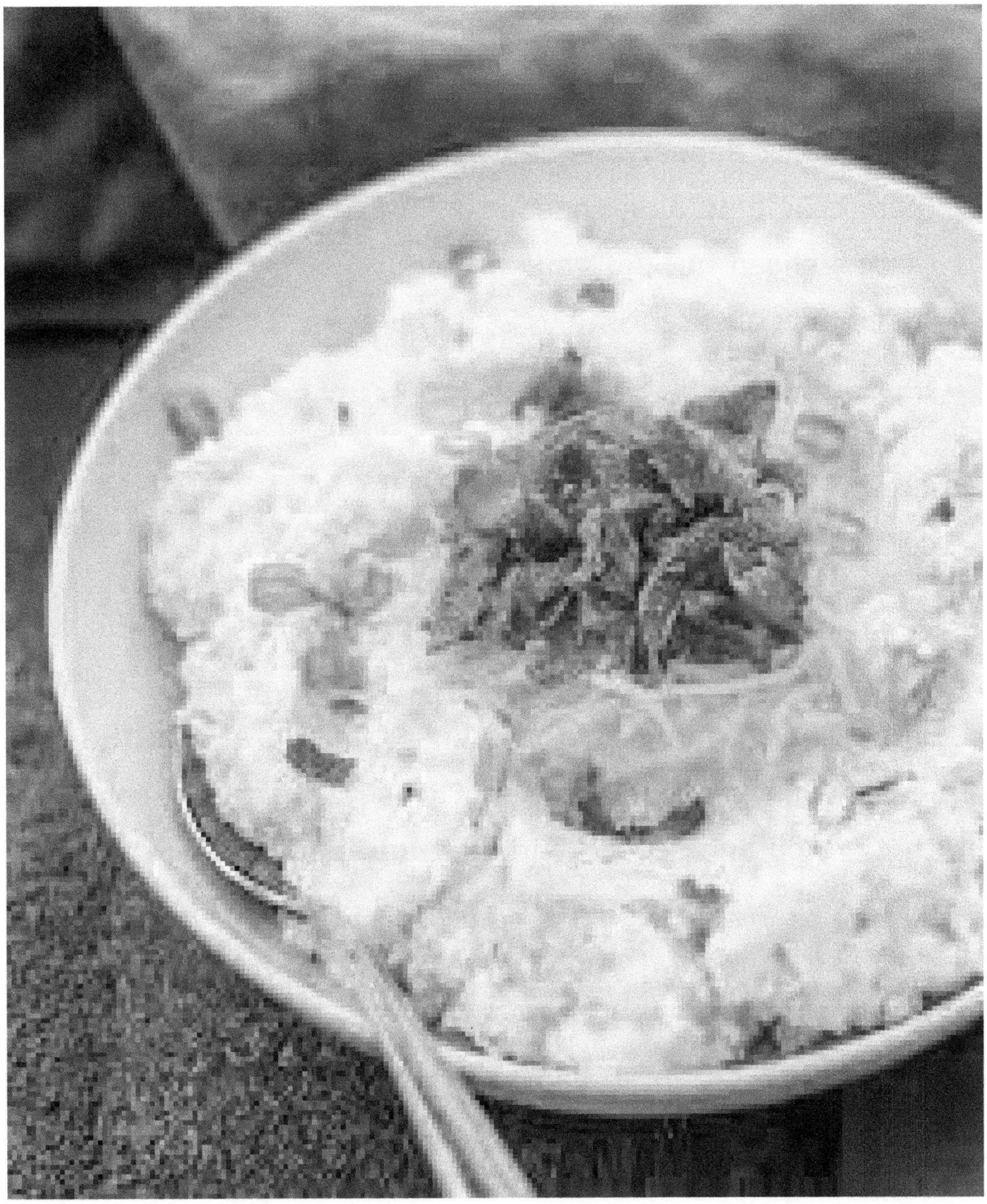

52 Spaghetti Squash With Blue Cheese And Bacon

(Ready in about 15 minutes | Serving 2 | Difficulty: Easy)

Per serving: Kcal 339, Fat: 24.3g, Sodium 691.2mg, Protein: 13.5g

Ingredients

- 1 tbsp. olive oil
- 1 spaghetti squash, small
- Ground black pepper and salt according to taste
- 2 tbsp. crumbled blue cheese
- 1 (4 oz.) sliced package mushrooms
- 4 slices bacon, diced into 1/2-inch pieces
- 1 clove minced garlic
- ¼ cup of sour cream
- 2 cup of baby spinach

Instruction

- Preheat oven to 400 degrees Fahrenheit. Aluminum foil can be used to line a baking sheet.
- Using a sharp knife, cut the stem from the end of the spaghetti squash. Squash can be cut in half lengthwise, and the seeds scraped off. Brush with olive oil and season with salt and pepper.
- Bake for forty-five minutes in a preheated oven till tender. Remove the fried flesh to a bowl and put it aside. Return the shells of the spaghetti squash to the baking sheet.
- Cook the bacon in a big skillet over medium-high flame, sometimes flipping, for five to six minutes, or till evenly browned. On paper towels, drain the bacon slices.
- Cook for four to five minutes with the garlic and mushrooms in the skillet. In a large mixing bowl, combine the spinach and cooked bacon. Stir for two to three minutes or till spinach is wilted. Toss the mushroom mixture

into the squash bowl. Combine the salt, pepper, and sour cream in a mixing bowl. Stir until all of the fillings are distributed.

- Fill the squash shells with the filling. On each half, sprinkle 1 tbsp. blue cheese. Return to oven and bake for another four to five minutes, or till the cheese has melted and the squash has cooked through.

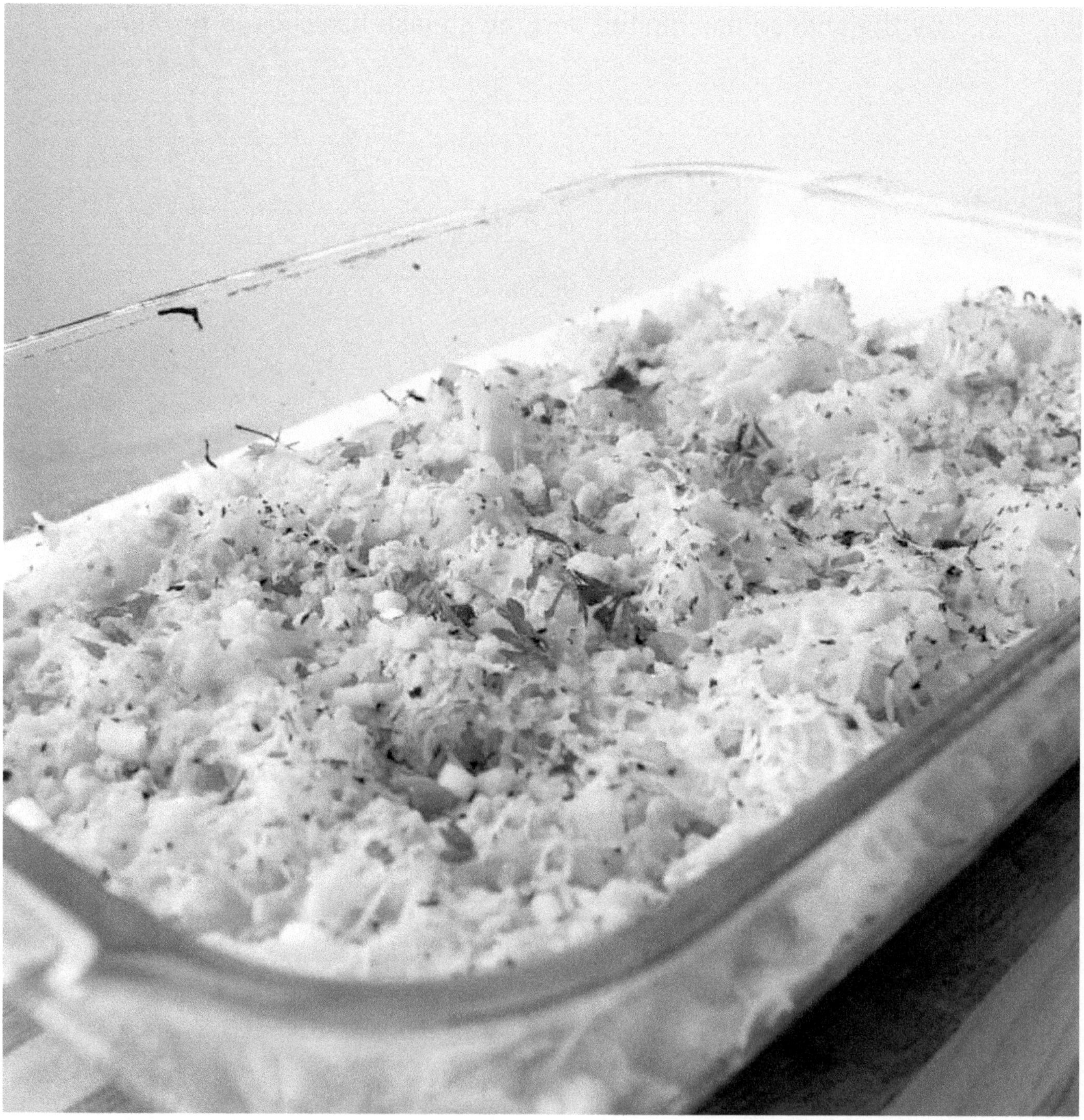

53 Ranch Cauliflower Crackers

(Ready in about 20 minutes | Serving 18 | Difficulty: Easy)

Per serving: Kcal 29, Fat: 1.5g, Sodium 103.5mg, Protein: 2.5g

Ingredients

- Cheesecloth
- 1 (12 oz.) frozen riced cauliflower
- 1 cup of Parmesan cheese, shredded
- 1 egg
- ⅛ tsp. cayenne pepper, or according to taste
- 1 tbsp. salad dressing mix, dry ranch

Instructions

- In a microwave-safe bowl, put the riced cauliflower. Microwave for three to four minutes, covered. Allow it to cool for fifteen minutes in a strainer lined with cheesecloth. Squeeze the moisture out of the riced cauliflower after it has cooled.
- Preheat oven to 425 degrees Fahrenheit. Using parchment paper, line the baking dish.
- In a mixing bowl, combine the egg, riced cauliflower, cayenne pepper, and ranch blend. Stir in the Parmesan cheese till it is fully incorporated.
- With a tiny cookie scoop, transfer the mixture onto a prepared cookie sheet and flatten it to around 1/16-inch thickness with a tiny hand-rolling pin, cup, or your hand. The crispier your cracker is, the thinner the dough will be.
- Bake for ten minutes in a preheated oven, then flip and bake for another ten minutes. Allow cooling on a wire shelf.

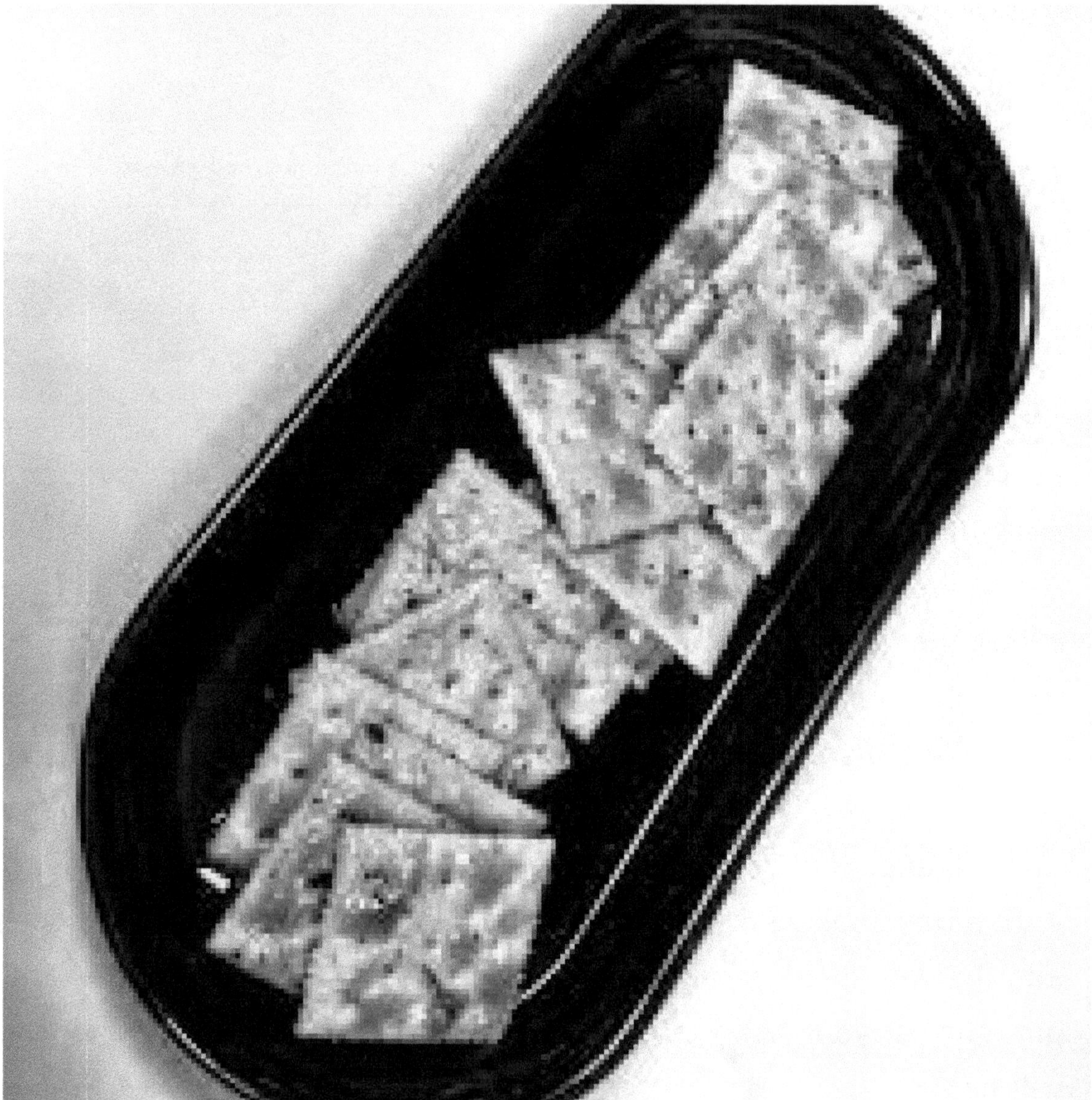

54 Easy Cauliflower Casserole

(Ready in about 10 minutes | Serving 2 | Difficulty: Easy)

Per serving: Kcal 469, Fat: 40.9g, Sodium 494.1mg, Protein: 18.1g

Ingredients

- 1 cup of Cheddar cheese, shredded
- ½ head cauliflower florets
- 1 pinch freshly ground black pepper and salt or according to taste
- ½ cup of heavy cream

Instruction

- Preheat oven to 400 degrees Fahrenheit.
- Cook the cauliflower in a big pot of lightly salted water until soft yet firm to the bite, approximately ten minutes. Drain.
- In a big mixing bowl, combine the cream, Cheddar cheese, pepper, and salt. Cover cauliflower with the cheese mixture in a casserole dish.
- Bake for twenty-five minutes in a preheated oven till the cheese is golden brown and bubbly.

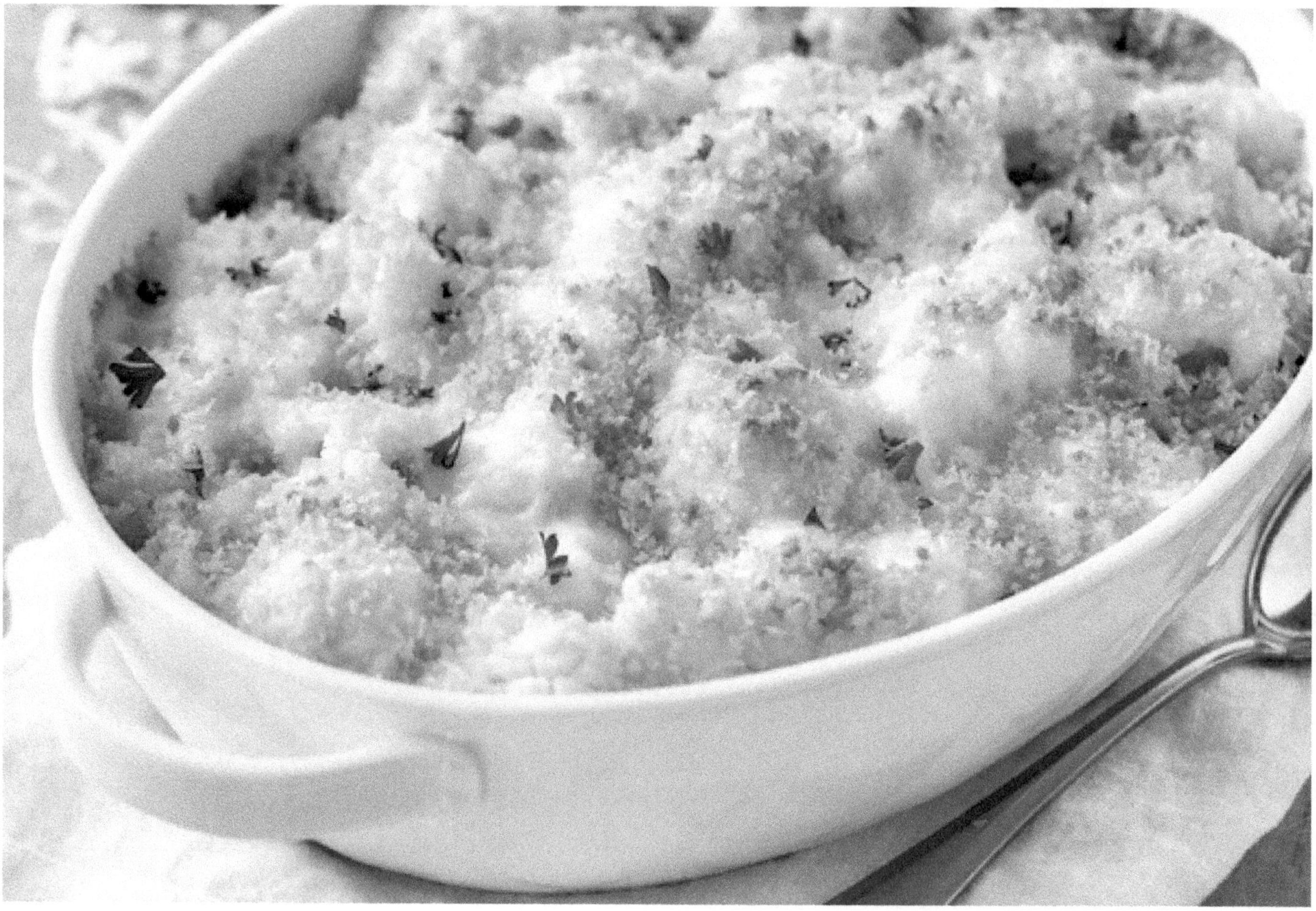

55 White Chicken Chili

(Ready in about 20 minutes | Serving 8 | Difficulty: Easy)

Per serving: Kcal 591, Fat: 49.6g, Sodium 795mg, Protein: 31.8g

Ingredients

- 1 stick divide butter
- 1 tbsp. oil, or as required
- 2 lb. Boneless, skinless, chicken breasts
- Ground black pepper and salt according to taste
- 1 ½ tsp. chili powder
- ¾ cup of chicken broth
- 4 oz. cream cheese
- 2 cup of heavy whipping cream
- 1 ½ tbsp. onion powder
- 1 tsp. hot sauce
- 2 tsp. cumin
- 2 (4 oz.) cans green chilies, chopped
- 1 ½ cup of Monterey Jack cheese, grated

Instruction

- Add oil and two tbsp. Butter to a big skillet and cook over medium-high flame.
- Season the chicken with salt, black pepper, and chili powder in the meantime. Cook the chicken in skillet for five minutes, on the one hand, resisting the temptation to turn it too soon. Cook, sometimes flipping to avoid burning, until the insides are no longer pink and the juices run free, approximately ten to fifteen minutes, relying on thickness. Transfer the chicken to the plate to cool for ten minutes or before it is ready to handle. Set aside chicken that has been shredded with your fingertips.

- In a big, heavy pot, combine the remaining 6 tbsp. Butter, heavy cream, chicken broth, cream cheese, cumin, hot sauce, and onion powder. Season with the black pepper and salt, then reduce to low heat and cook for five minutes, or until the butter and cream cheese have melted.
- To the chili in a pot, add shredded chicken, Monterey Jack cheese, and green chiles. Reduce the heat to low and simmer for twenty minutes, stirring occasionally.

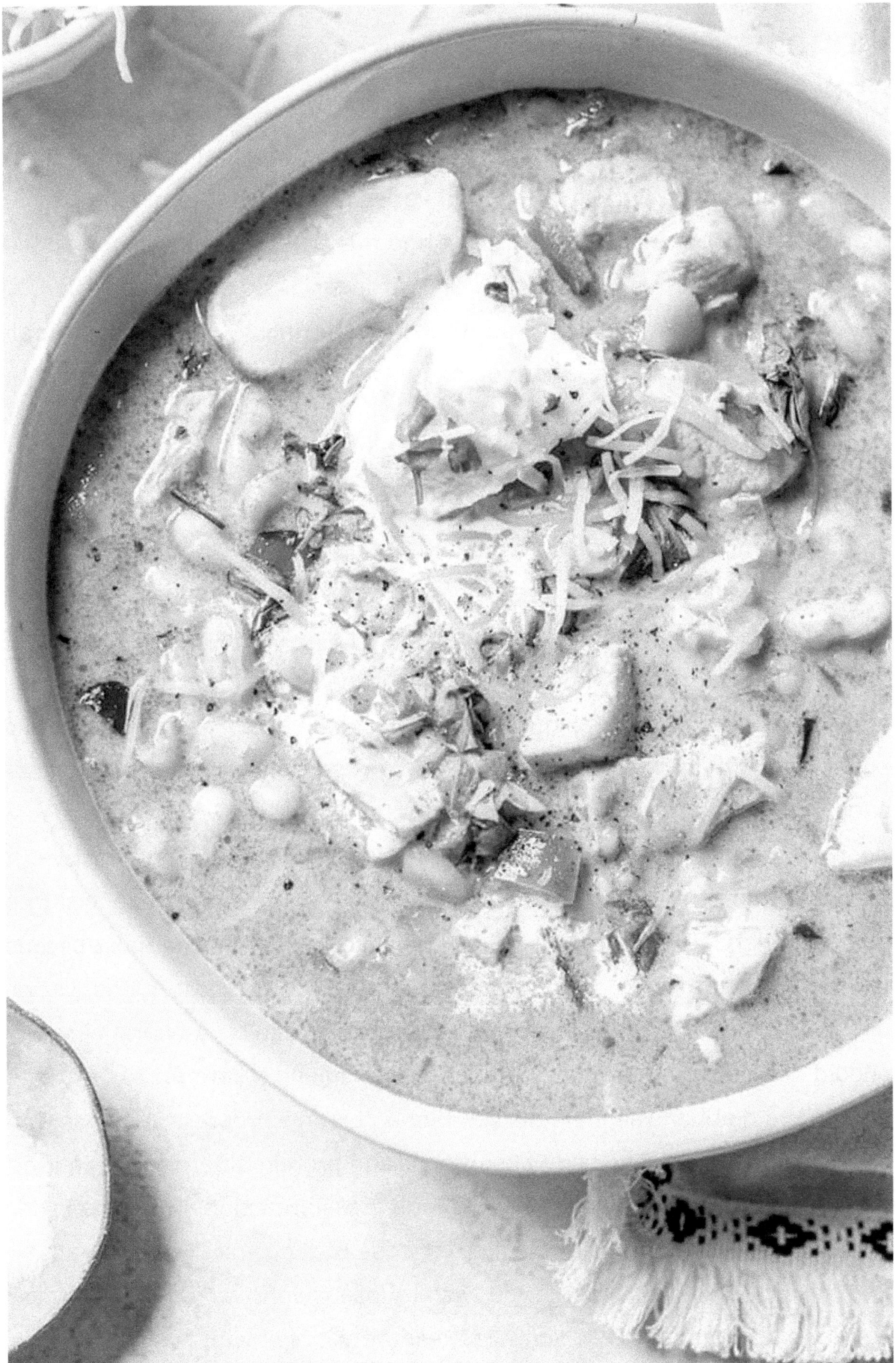

Conclusion

A keto diet may be a healthier option for certain people, although the amount of fat, carbohydrates, and protein prescribed varies from person to person. If you have diabetes, talk to the doctor before starting the diet because it would almost certainly need prescription changes and stronger blood sugar regulation. Are you taking drugs for high blood pressure? Before starting a keto diet again, talk to the doctor. If you're breastfeeding, you shouldn't follow a ketogenic diet. Be mindful that limiting carbs will render you irritable, hungry, and sleepy, among other things. However, this may be a one-time occurrence. Keep in mind that you can eat a balanced diet in order to obtain all of the vitamins and minerals you need. A sufficient amount of fiber is also needed. When the body begins to derive energy from accumulated fat rather than glucose, it is said to be in ketosis. Several trials have shown the powerful weight-loss benefits of a low-carb, or keto, diet. This diet, on the other hand, can be difficult to stick to and can exacerbate health issues in individuals who have certain disorders, such as diabetes type 1. The keto diet is suitable for the majority of citizens. Nonetheless, all major dietary modifications should be discussed with a dietitian or doctor. This is essentially the case with people who have inherent conditions. The keto diet may be an effective therapy for people with drug-resistant epilepsy. Though the diet may be beneficial to people of any age, teenagers, people over 50, and babies can profit the most because they can easily stick to it. Modified keto diets, such as the revised Atkins diet or the low-glycemic index diet, are safer for adolescents and adults. A health care worker should keep a careful eye on someone who is taking a keto diet as a treatment. A doctor and dietitian will maintain track of a person's progress, administer drugs, and test for side effects. The body absorbs fat and protein differently than it does carbohydrates. Carbohydrates have a high insulin reaction. The protein sensitivity to insulin is mild, and the quick insulin response is negligible. Insulin is a fat-producing and fat-conserving enzyme. If you wish to lose weight, consume as many eggs, chickens, fish, and birds as you want, satiate yourself with the fat, and then eat every vegetable that grows on the ground. Butter and coconut oil can be used instead of processed synthetic seed oils. You may be either a sugar or a fat burner, but not both.

Keto Chaffle Cookbook

An Easy Guide to Make Delicious Chaffles with Low Carb Recipes to Lose Weight, Improve Your Health and Satisfy your soul. With Pictures!

By

Camila Rivera

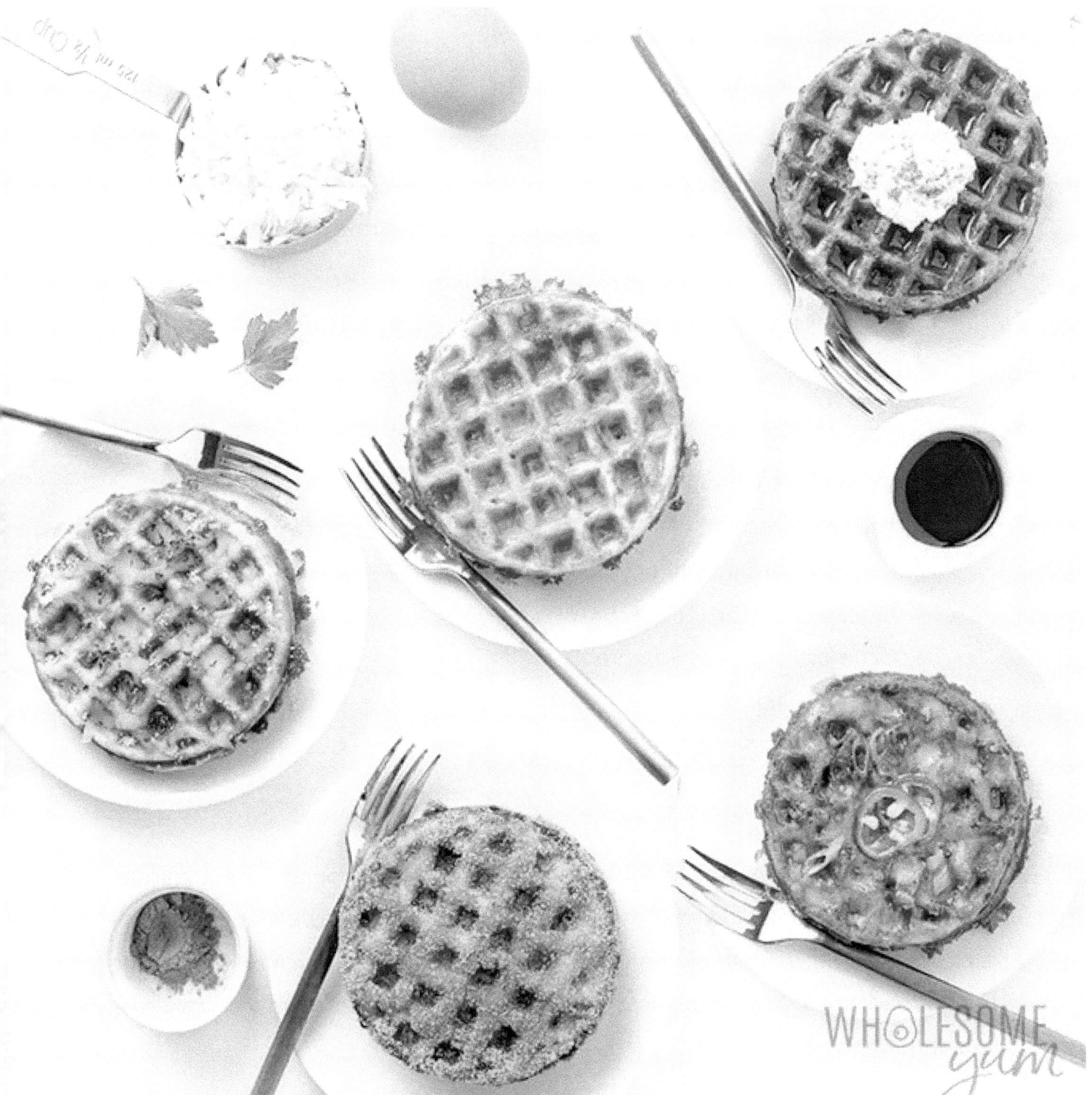
WHOLESOME yum

Keto Chaffle Recipes

1 Oreo Chaffles

(Ready in about 23 minutes | Serving 2 | Difficulty: Easy)

Per serving: Kcal 1381, Fat: 146g, Net Carbs: 14g, Protein: 17g

Ingredients

- 1/2 cup of Sugar-Free Chocolate Chips
- 1 tsp of Vanilla extract
- 3 Eggs
- 1/2 cup of butter
- 1/4 cup of sweetener

Cheese Frosting

- 4 ounces of Cream Cheese
- 4 ounces of butter
- 1/2 cup of Powdered Swerve
- 1 tsp of Vanilla extract
- 1/4 cup of Whipping Cream

Instructions

Melt chocolate and butter in a bowl in the microwave for around 1 minute. Stir to remove clumps. Mix vanilla, egg and sweetener in a bowl. Pour a quarter of the mixture into the waffle maker and cook for around 8 minutes. Mix frosting ingredients in the food processor's bowl in the meantime and make a smooth mixture. Spread frosting among two chaffles.

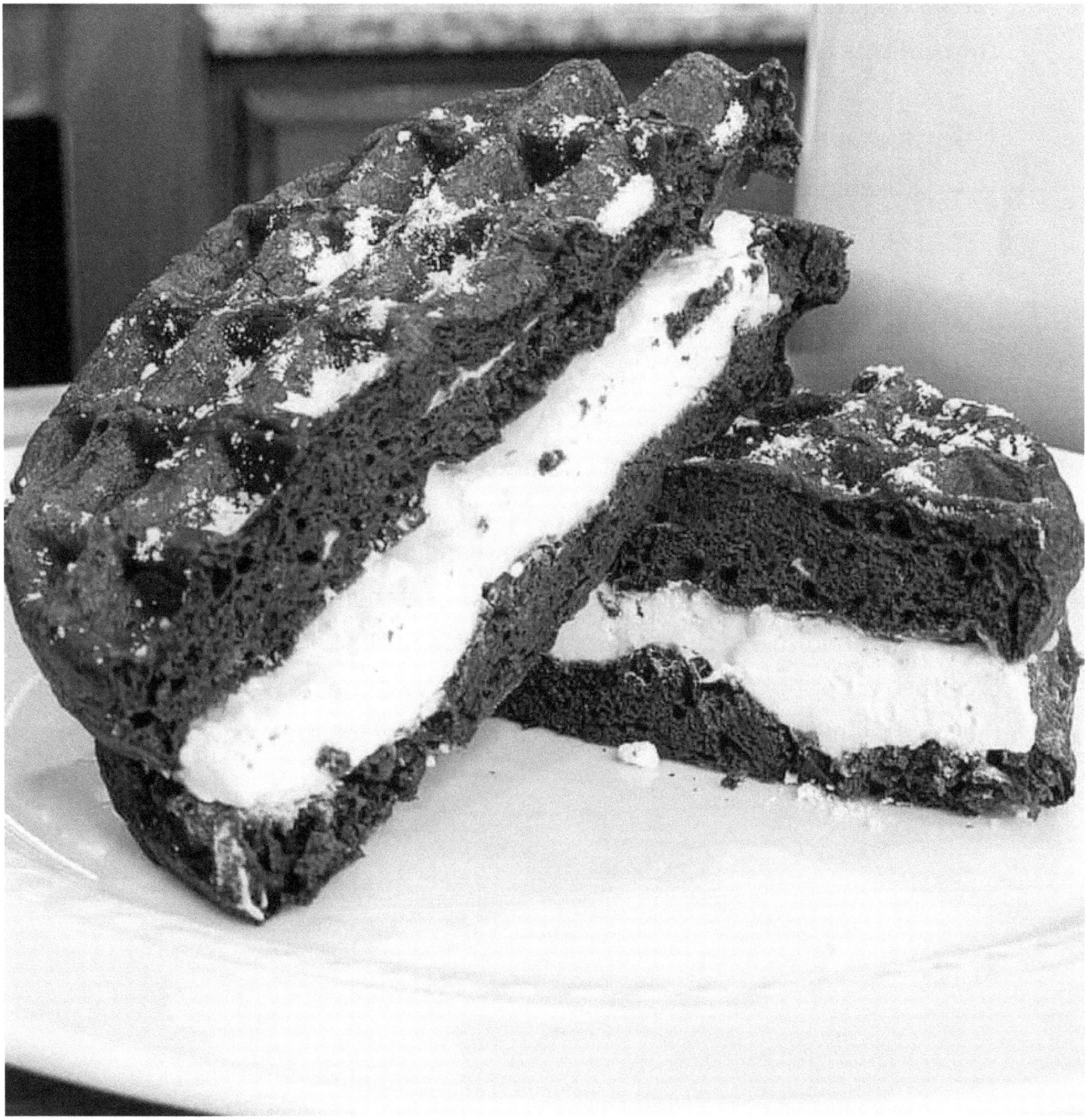

2 Strawberry Chaffles

(Ready in about 35 minutes | Serving 8 | Difficulty: Moderate)

Per serving: Kcal 189, Fat: 14.3g, Net Carbs: 5.2g, Protein: 10g

Ingredients

- 3 oz of cream cheese
- 1 cup of whipped cream
- 2 beaten eggs
- 2 cups shredded mozzarella cheese
- 1/2 cup of almond flour
- 2 tsp of baking powder
- 3 tbsp of sweetener
- 8 strawberries
- 1 tbsp of sweetener

Instructions

Add mozzarella and cream cheese to a bowl and microwave for around 1 minute. Beat eggs and mix with baking powder, 3 tbsp sweetener and almond flour. Mix it with cheese and add to 2 diced strawberries. Place in the fridge for around 20 minutes. Dice the rest of the strawberries and add tbsp sweetener. Warm waffle iron and add the quarter mixture from the fridge to the center of the iron. Cook for around 7 minutes.

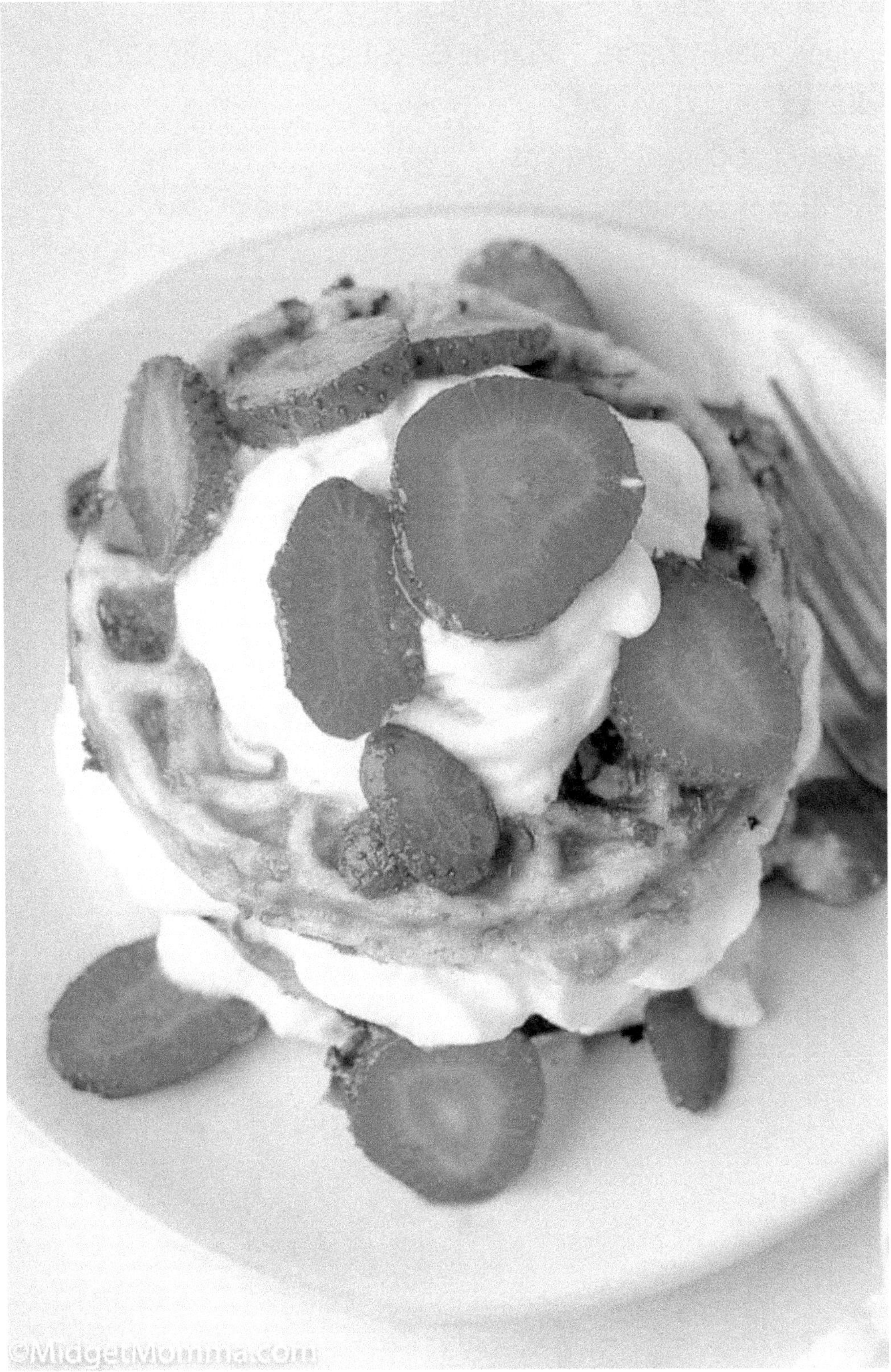
©MidgetMomma.com

3 Chocolate Chaffle

(Ready in about 18 minutes | Serving 2 | Difficulty: Easy)

Per serving: Kcal 672, Fat: 70g, Net Carbs: 11g, Protein: 13g

Ingredients

- 1/2 cup of Chocolate Chips
- 1/4 cup of sweetener
- 3 Eggs
- 1/2 cup of butter
- 1 tsp of Vanilla extract

Instructions

Melt chocolate and butter in a bowl in the microwave for around 1 minute. Stir and remove clumps. Blend sweetener, vanilla and eggs in a bowl. Add chocolate and butter and whisk. Pour the quarter amount of mixture into a waffle maker. Cook for around 8 minutes.

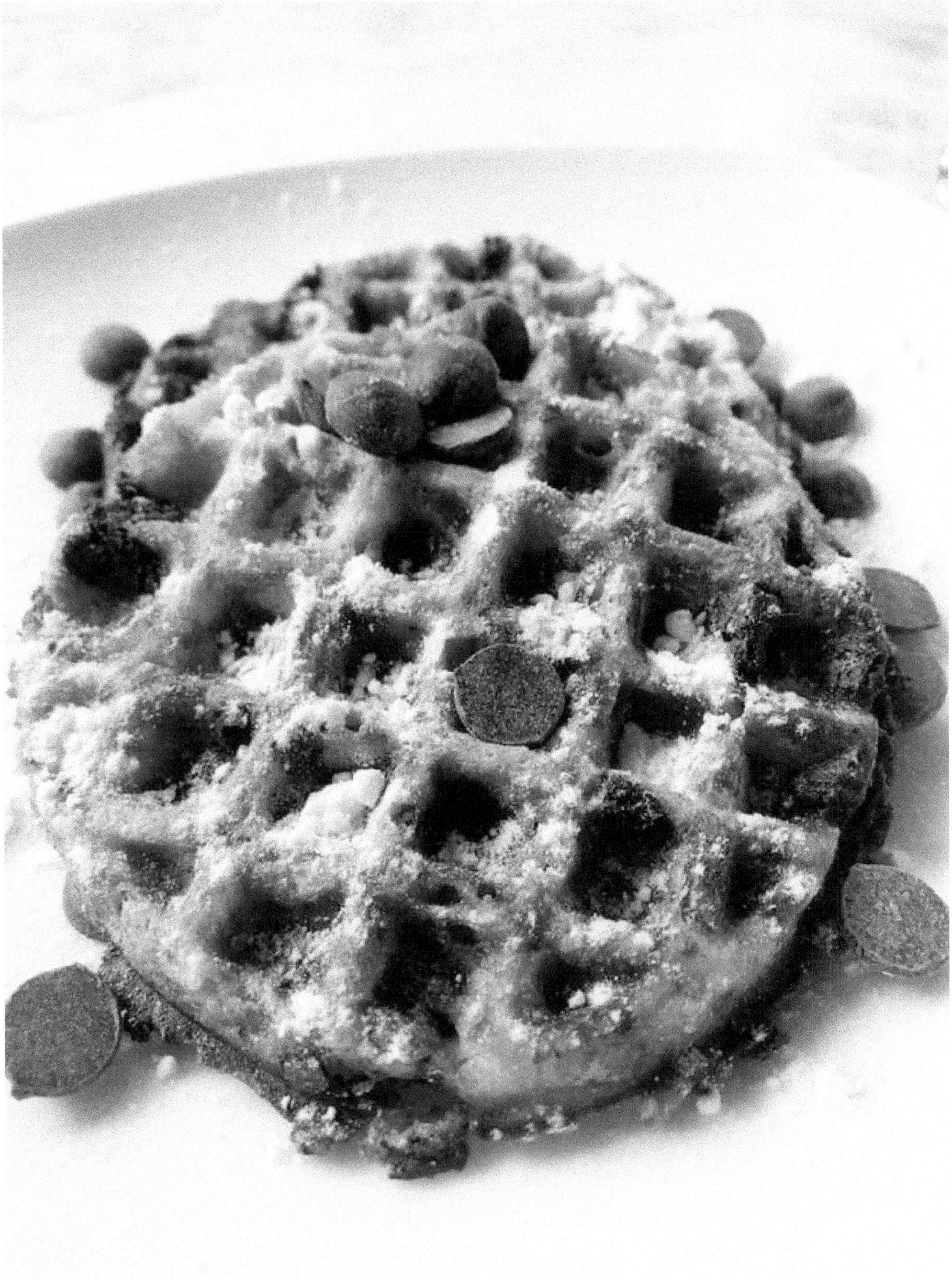

4 Pumpkin Chaffles

(Ready in about 7 minutes | Serving 1 | Difficulty: Easy)

Per serving: Kcal 250, Fat: 15g, Net Carbs: 5g, Protein: 23g

Ingredients

- 1/2 cup mozzarella cheese shredded
- 1 1/2tbsp of pumpkin purée
- 1 beaten egg
- 1/2tsp of Swerve confectioners
- 1/4tsp of Pumpkin Pie Spice
- 1/2tsp of vanilla extract
- ⅛ tsp of maple extract

Instructions

Mix all the ingredients except mozzarella cheese in a bowl and mix. Add cheese and whisk. Spray waffle using cooking spray. Place half amount of batter in the center of the waffle maker. Cook for around 6 minutes. Repeat with the remaining batter.

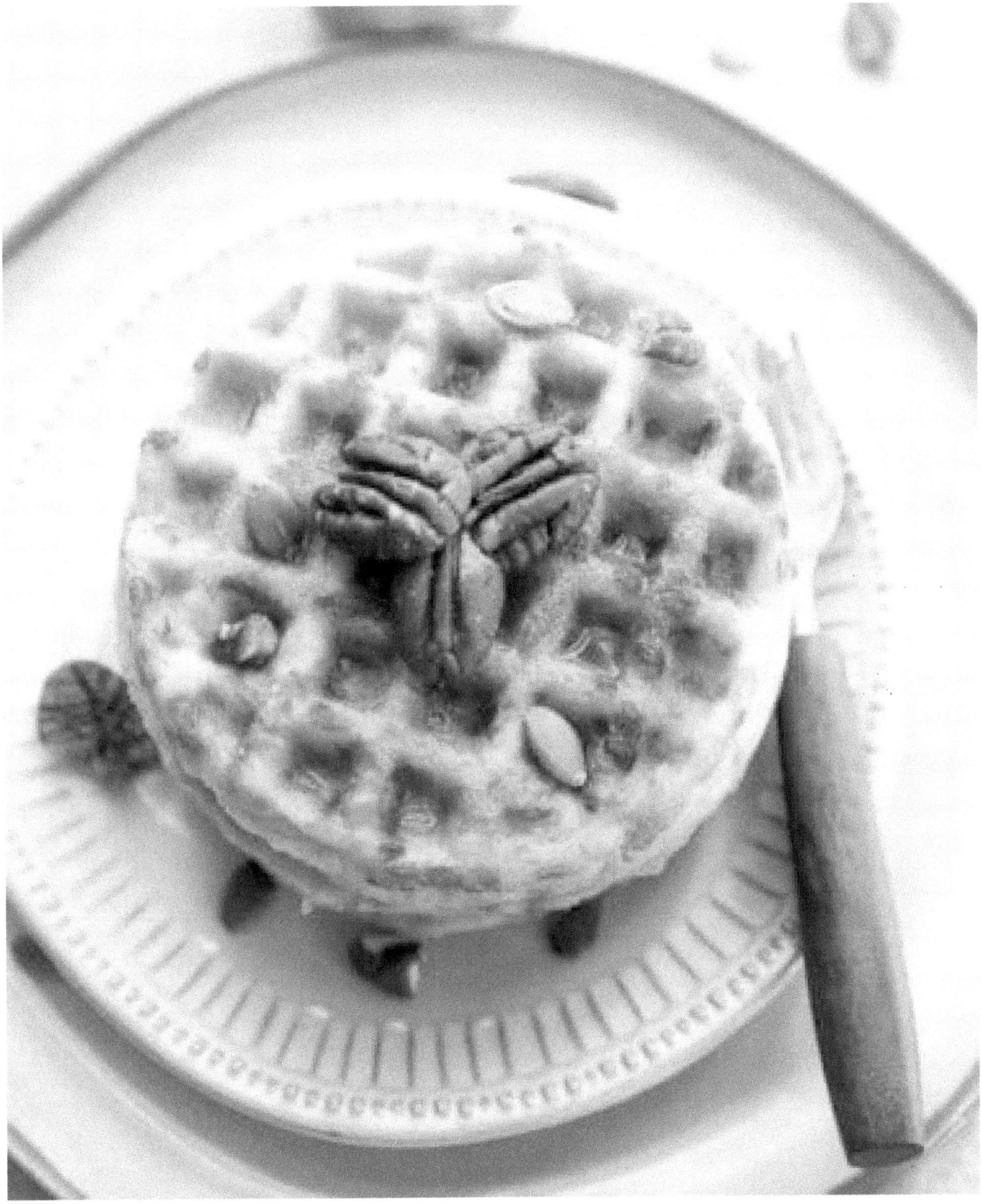

5 Basic Chaffle

(Ready in about 8 minutes | Serving 2 | Difficulty: Easy)

Per serving: Kcal 208, Fat: 16g, Net Carbs: 4g, Protein: 11g

Ingredients

- 1 Big Egg
- 2 tbsp of Almond Flour
- 1/2 cup shredded Mozzarella cheese

Instructions

Preheat waffle iron for around 5 minutes. Microwave cheese for around 30 seconds. Add the rest of the ingredients and mix. Pour mixture that covers the surface of the waffle maker. Cook for around 4 minutes. Take out and place on a plate and repeat with the rest of the batter.

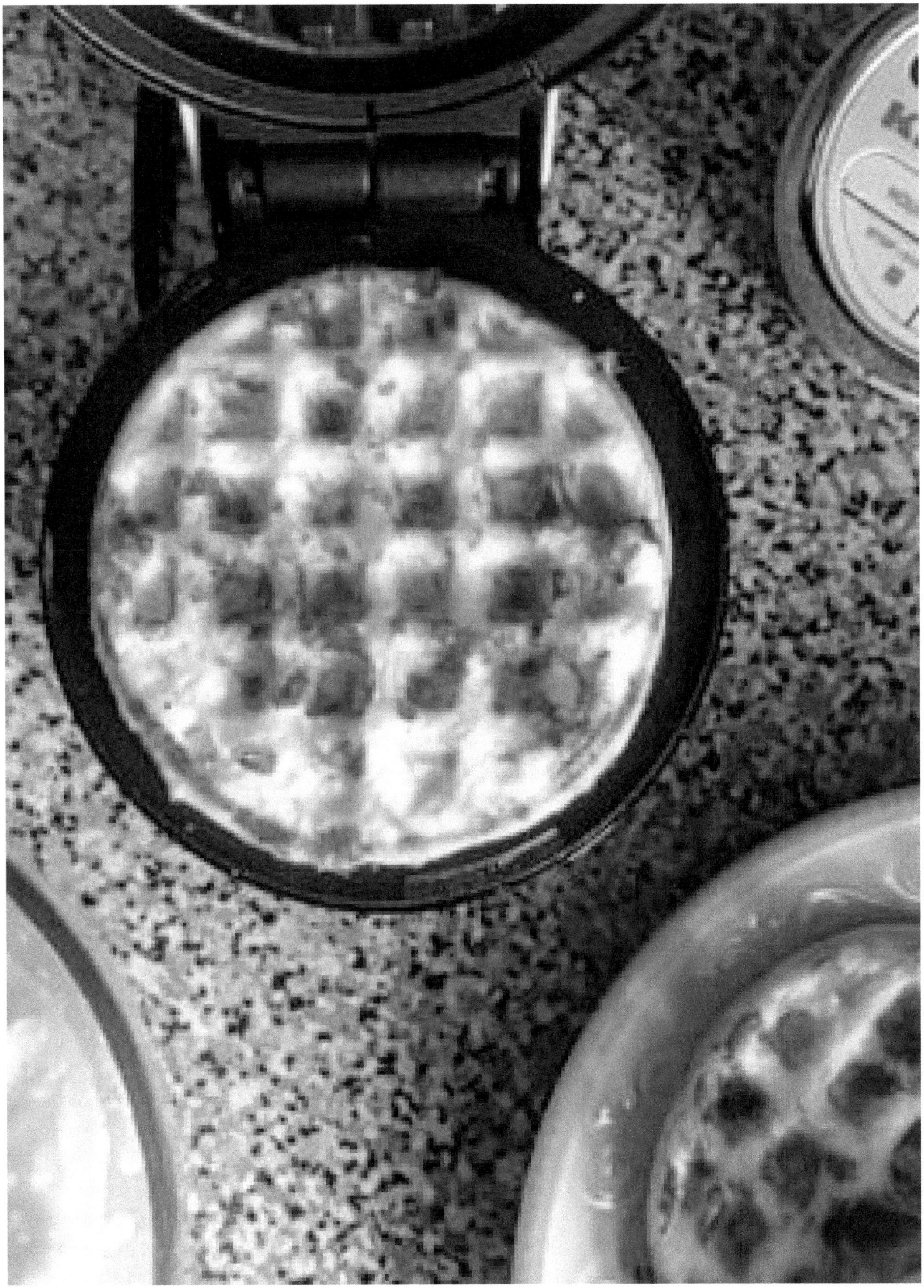

6 Garlic Chaffles

(Ready in about 8 minutes | Serving 2 | Difficulty: Easy)

Per serving: Kcal 208, Fat: 16g, Net Carbs: 4g, Protein: 11g

Ingredients

- 1/3 cup Parmesan cheese Grated
- 1/2 cup shredded Mozzarella cheese
- 1 Big Egg
- 1/2 tsp of Italian seasoning
- 1 minced Garlic clove

Instructions

Preheat waffle iron for around 5 minutes. Microwave cream cheese for around 30 seconds. Add the rest of the ingredients except the toppings. Pour mixture that covers the surface of the waffle maker. Cook for around 4 minutes. Take out and place on a plate and repeat with the rest of the batter.

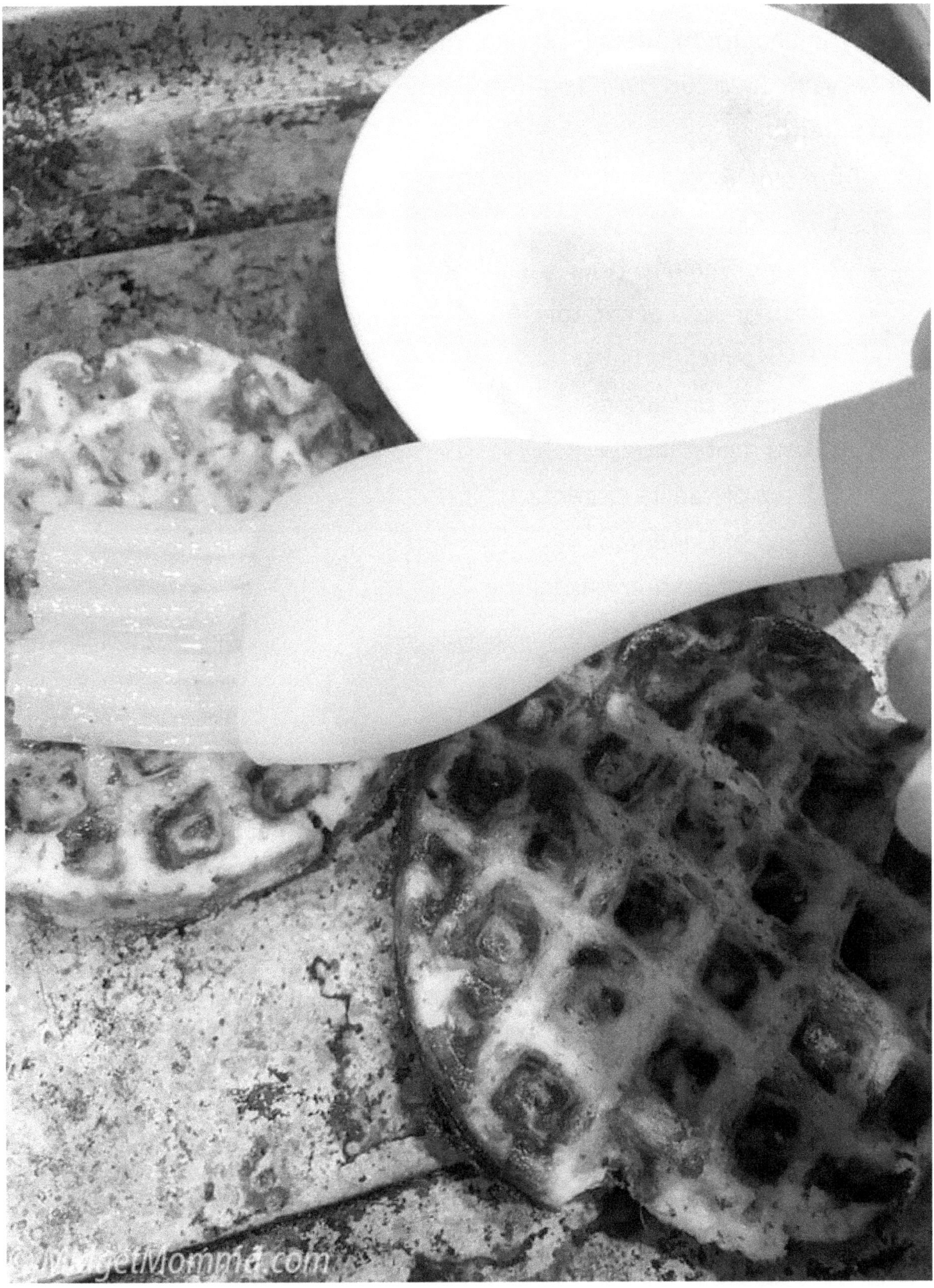
©MidgetMomma.com

7 Cinnamon Chaffles

(Ready in about 8 minutes | Serving 2 | Difficulty: Easy)

Per serving: Kcal 208, Fat: 16g, Net Carbs: 4g, Protein: 11g

Ingredients

- 3/4 cup shredded Mozzarella cheese
- 1 Big Egg
- 2 tbsp of Almond Flour
- 2 tbsp of besti erythritol
- 1/2 tbsp melted butter
- 1/2 tsp of cinnamon
- 1 tbsp melted butter
- 1/2 tsp of vanilla extract
- 3/4 tsp of cinnamon
- 1/4 cup of besti erythritol

Instructions

Preheat waffle iron for around 5 minutes. Microwave cream cheese for around 30 seconds. Add the rest of the ingredients except the toppings. Pour mixture that covers the surface of the waffle maker. Cook for around 4 minutes. Take out and place on a plate and repeat with the rest of the batter. To prepare churro chaffles, mix cinnamon and erythritol for topping. Brush chaffles using butter after they are cooked and sprinkle with topping.

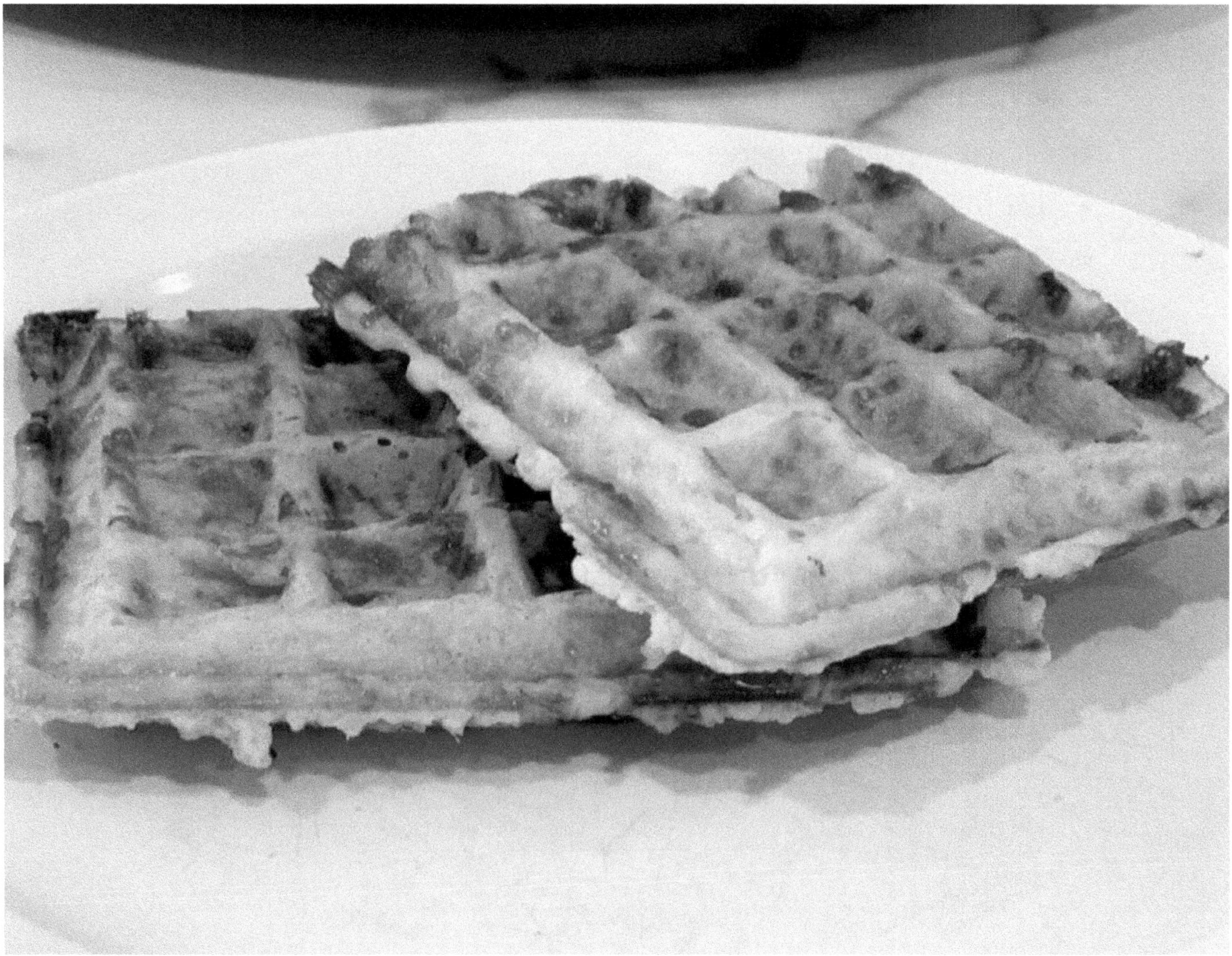

8 Cheese Chaffles

(Ready in about 8 minutes | Serving 2 | Difficulty: Easy)

Per serving: Kcal 208, Fat: 16g, Net Carbs: 4g, Protein: 11g

Ingredients

- 1 Egg
- 1/2 oz of Cream cheese
- 1/2 cup shredded Mozzarella cheese
- 2 1/2 tbsp of Besti Erythritol
- 2 tbsp of pumpkin puree
- 1/2 tbsp of Pumpkin pie spice
- 3 tsp of Coconut Flour

Instructions

Preheat waffle iron for around 5 minutes. Microwave cream cheese for around 30 seconds. Add the rest of the ingredients except the toppings. Pour mixture that covers the surface of the waffle maker. Cook for around 4 minutes. Take out and place on a plate and repeat with the rest of the batter.

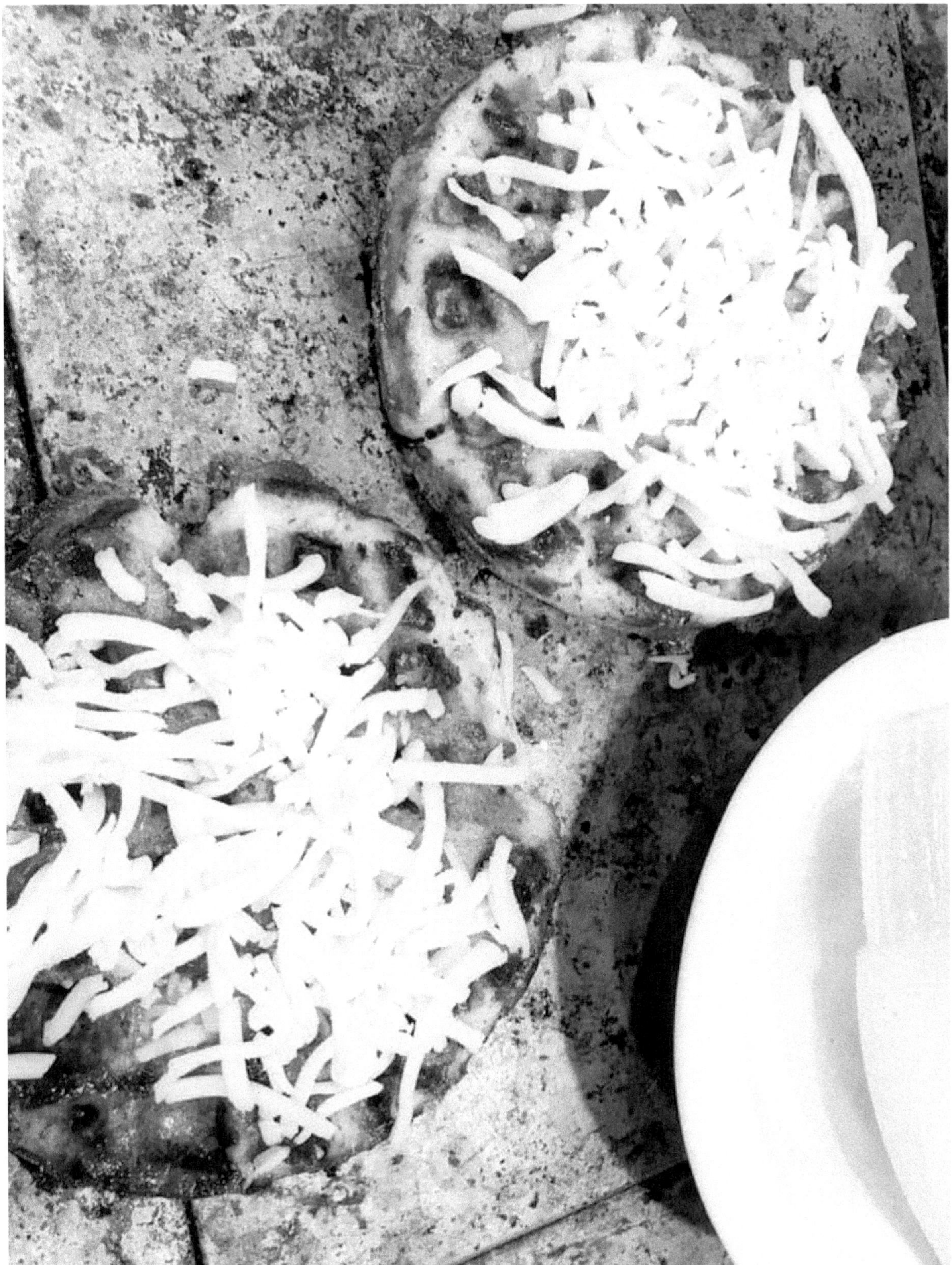
©MidgetMomma.com

9 Spicy Chaffles

(Ready in about 8 minutes | Serving 2 | Difficulty: Easy)

Per serving: Kcal 208, Fat: 16g, Net Carbs: 4g, Protein: 11g

Ingredients

- 1 Egg
- 1 oz of Cream cheese
- 1 cup shredded Cheddar cheese
- 1/2 tbsp of Jalapenos
- 2 tbsp of Bacon bits

Instructions

Preheat waffle iron for around 5 minutes. Microwave cream cheese for around 30 seconds. Add the rest of the ingredients except the toppings. Pour mixture that covers the surface of the waffle maker. Cook for around 4 minutes. Take out and place on a plate and repeat with the rest of the batter.

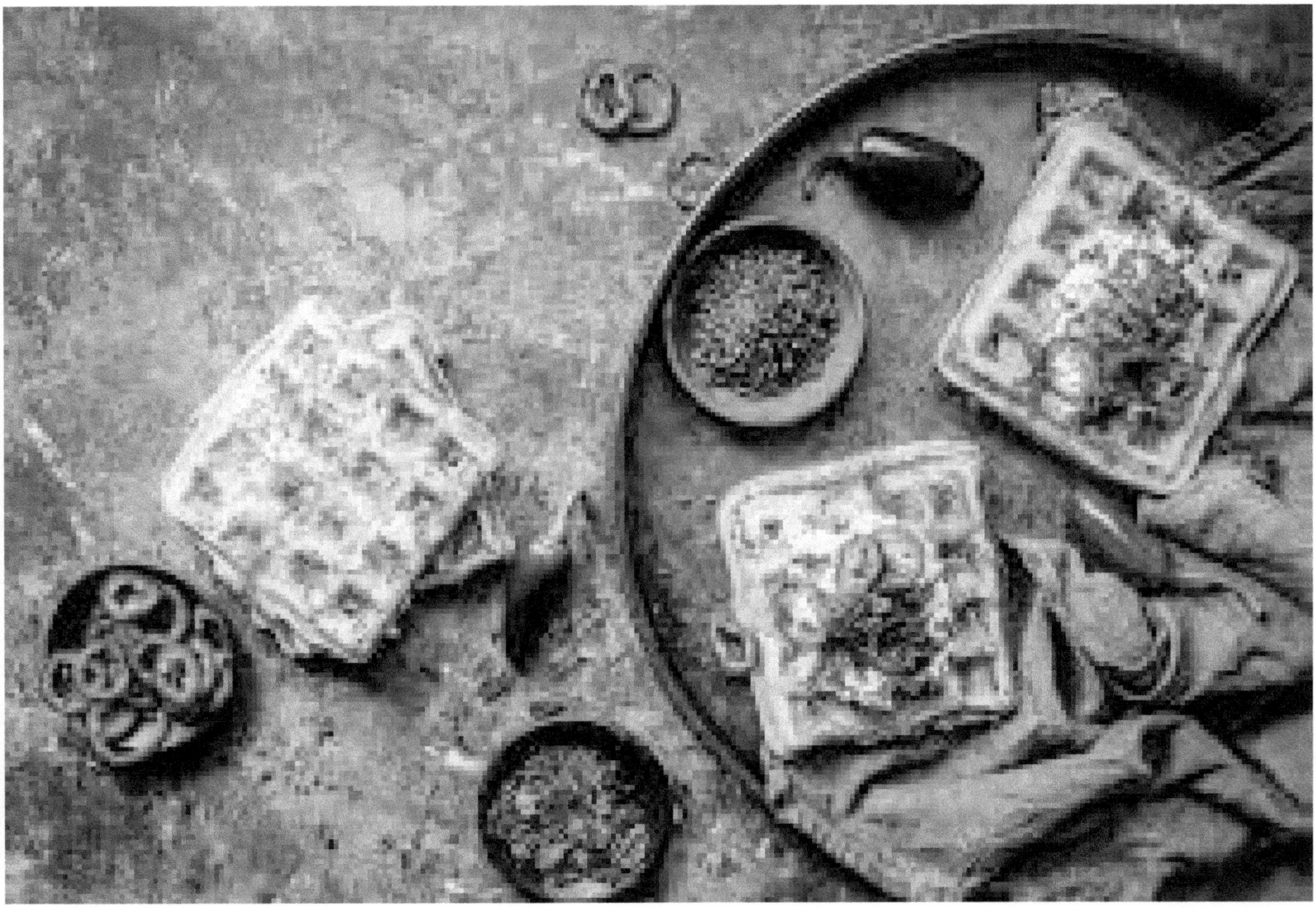

10 Double Chocolate Chaffles

(Ready in about 5 minutes | Serving 1 | Difficulty: Easy)

Per serving: Kcal 197, Fat: 23.3g, Net Carbs: 11.3g, Protein: 24.3g

Ingredients

- 1 egg
- 1 tbsp of granulated sweetener
- 1/2 cup grated mozzarella
- 1 tsp of vanilla
- 1 tbsp of chocolate chips
- 2 tbsp of almond meal/flour
- 1 tsp of heavy cream
- 2 tbsp unsweetened cocoa powder

Instructions

Add all the ingredients to a bowl and mix. Preheat the waffle maker. Spray with oil and pour half amount of batter into the maker. Cook for around 4 minutes. Sprinkle with toppings and enjoy.

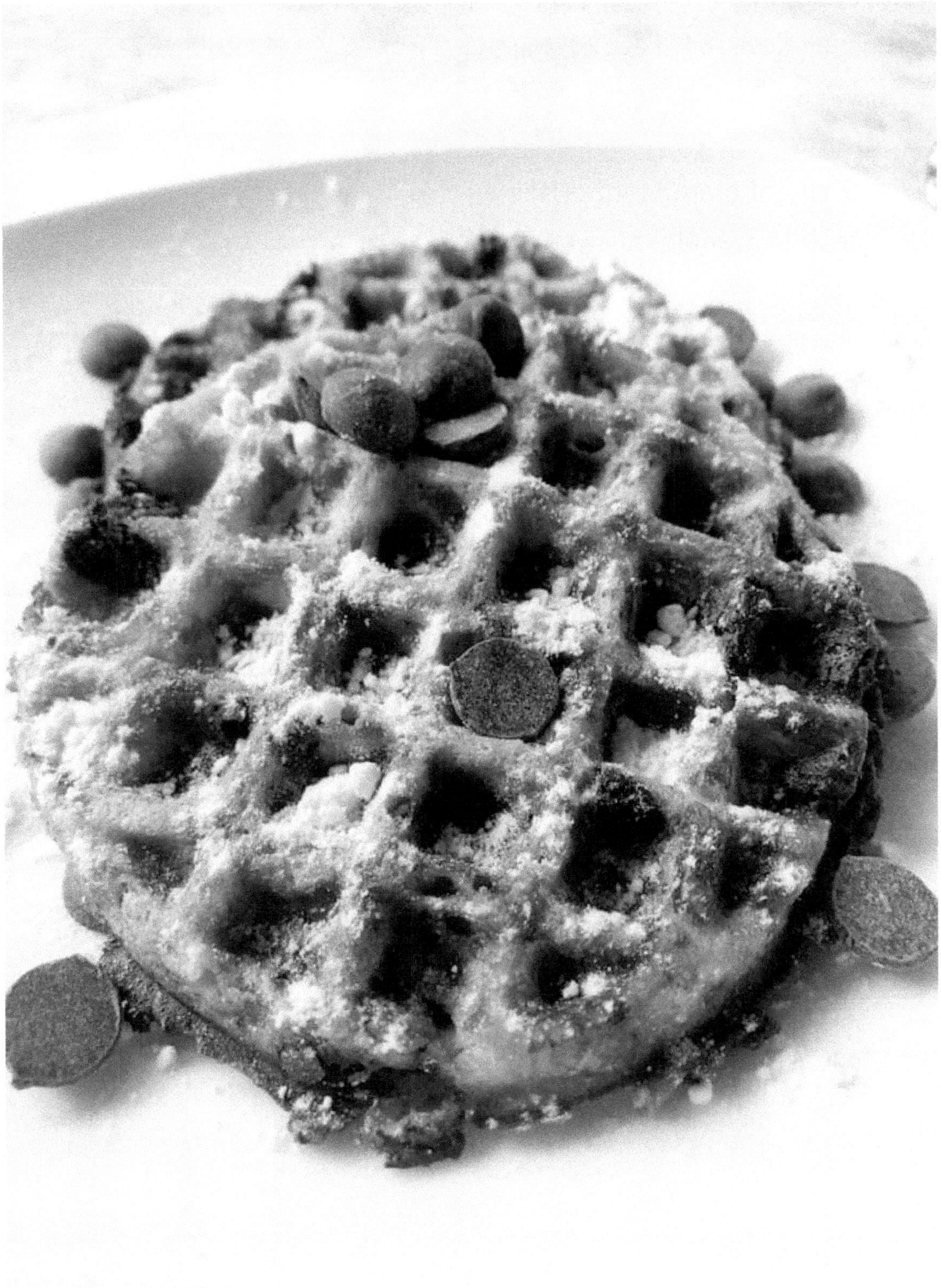

11 Vanilla Chaffles

(Ready in about 10 minutes | Serving 1 | Difficulty: Easy)

Per serving: Kcal 184, Fat: 20.1g, Net Carbs: 5.4g, Protein: 22.2g

Ingredients

- 1/2 cup of grated mozzarella
- 1 tbsp of granulated sweetener
- 1 eggs
- 1 tsp of vanilla extract
- 1 tbsp of chocolate chips
- 2 tbsp of almond flour

Instructions

Combine all the ingredients in a bowl. Preheat the waffle maker and spray it using oil once it is hot. Pour half amount of batter in the maker and cook for around 4 minutes. Remove and do the same with the rest of the batter. Top and enjoy.

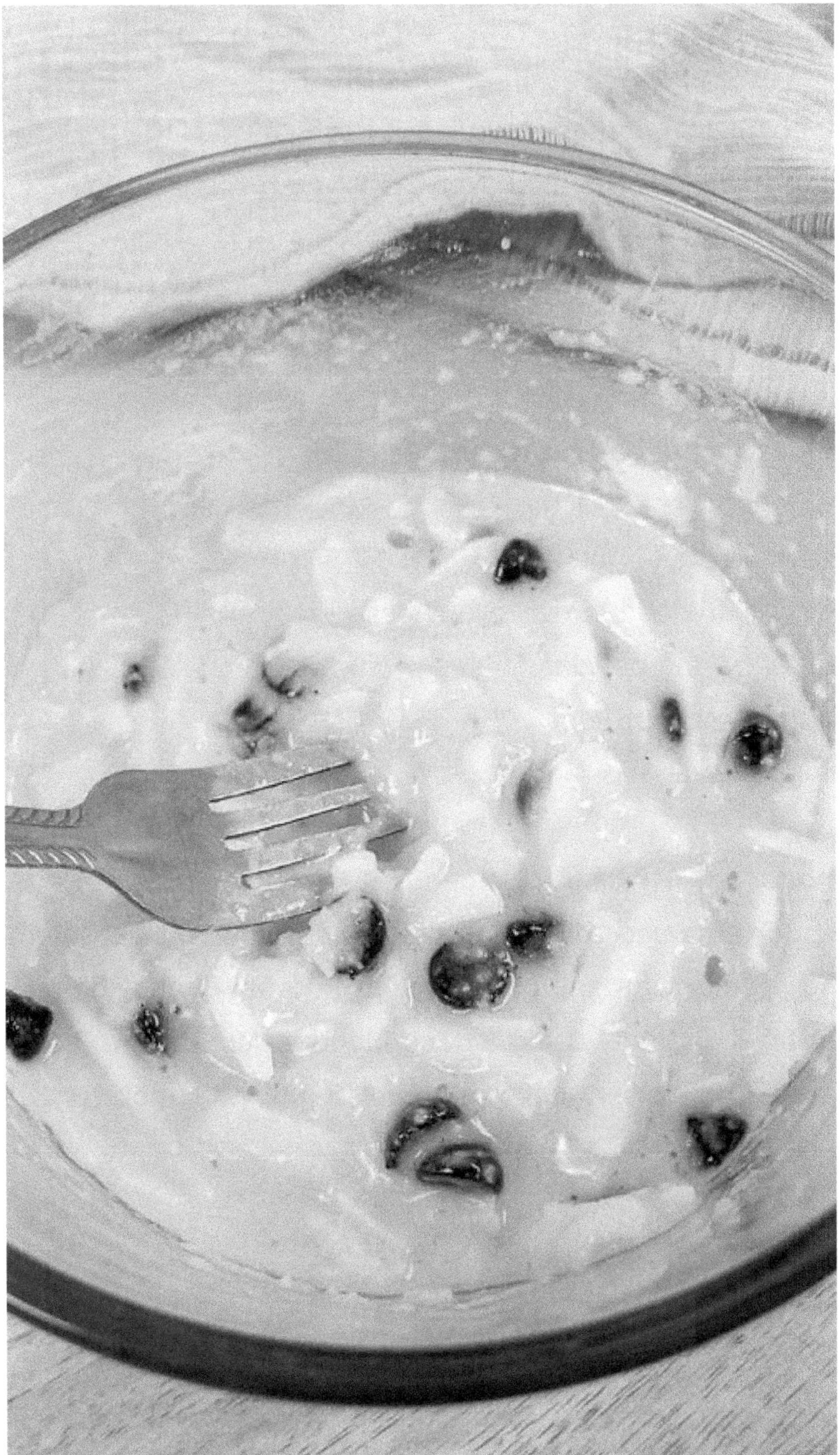
ditchthecarbs.com

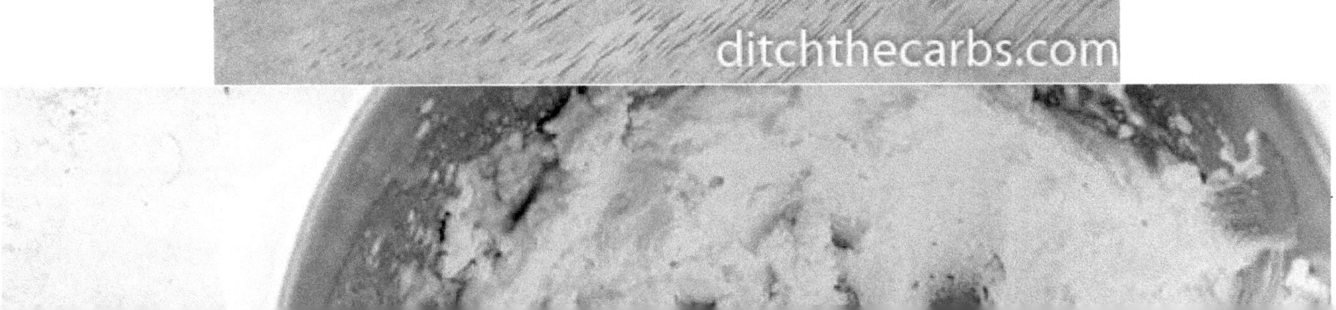

12 Lemon Curd Chaffle

(Ready in about 50 minutes | Serving 3 | Difficulty: Hard)

Per serving: Kcal 302, Fat: 24g, Net Carbs: 6g, Protein: 15g

Ingredients

- 3 eggs
- one batch of lemon curd
- 4 ounces softened cream cheese
- 1 tsp of vanilla extract
- 1 tbsp sweetener low carb
- 3/4 cup shredded mozzarella cheese
- 1 tsp of baking powder
- 3 tbsp of coconut flour
- 1/3 tsp of salt

Instructions

Prepare lemon curd according to package instructions. Heat the maker and spray oil. Mix baking powder, salt and coconut flour in a bowl. Add the rest of the ingredients to another bowl and beat using a hand blender. Mix the two bowls mixture and pour in the maker. Cook for around 5 minutes. Top using lemon curd.

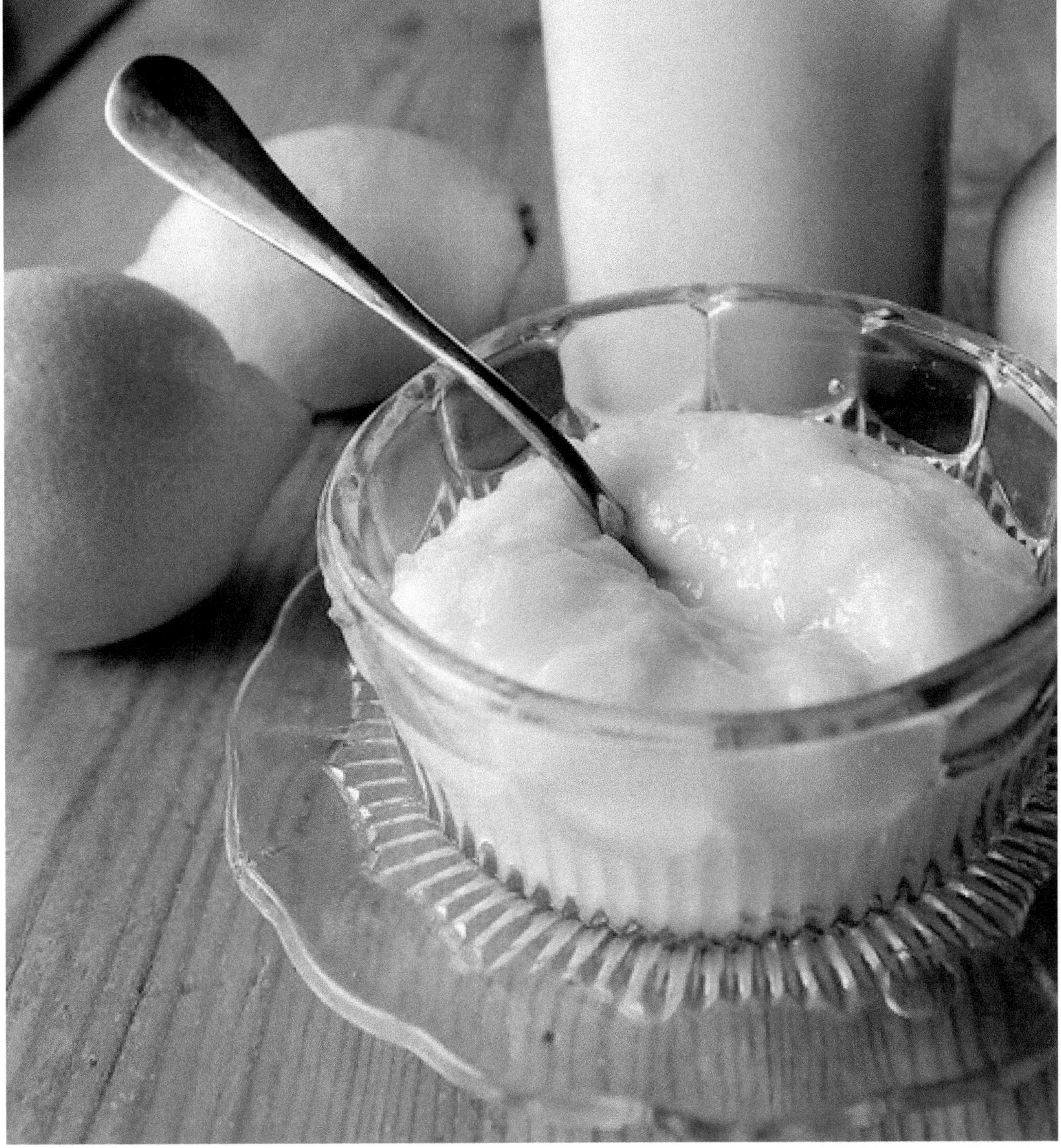

13 Glazed Donut

(Ready in about 15 minutes | Serving 3 | Difficulty: Easy)

Per serving: Kcal 246, Fat: 17g, Net Carbs: 2g, Protein: 14g

Ingredients

For chaffles

- 1/2 cup shredded cheese Mozzarella
- 2 tbsp of whey protein
- 1 ounce of Cream Cheese
- 2 tbsp of Swerve confectioners
- 1/2tsp of Vanilla extract
- 1/2tsp of Baking powder
- 1 Egg

For glaze

- 1/2tsp of Vanilla extract
- 3-4 tbsp of Swerve confectioners
- 2 tbsp of whipping cream

Instructions

Preheat the waffle maker. Add cream cheese and mozzarella in a bowl and microwave for around 30 seconds. Add 2 tbsp sweetener, whey protein and baking powder and mix. Add dough to a bowl and break an egg into it and add vanilla. Stir to form a smooth mixture. Add batter to the waffle maker and cook for around 5 minutes. Beat glaze ingredients in a bowl and top chaffles with it.

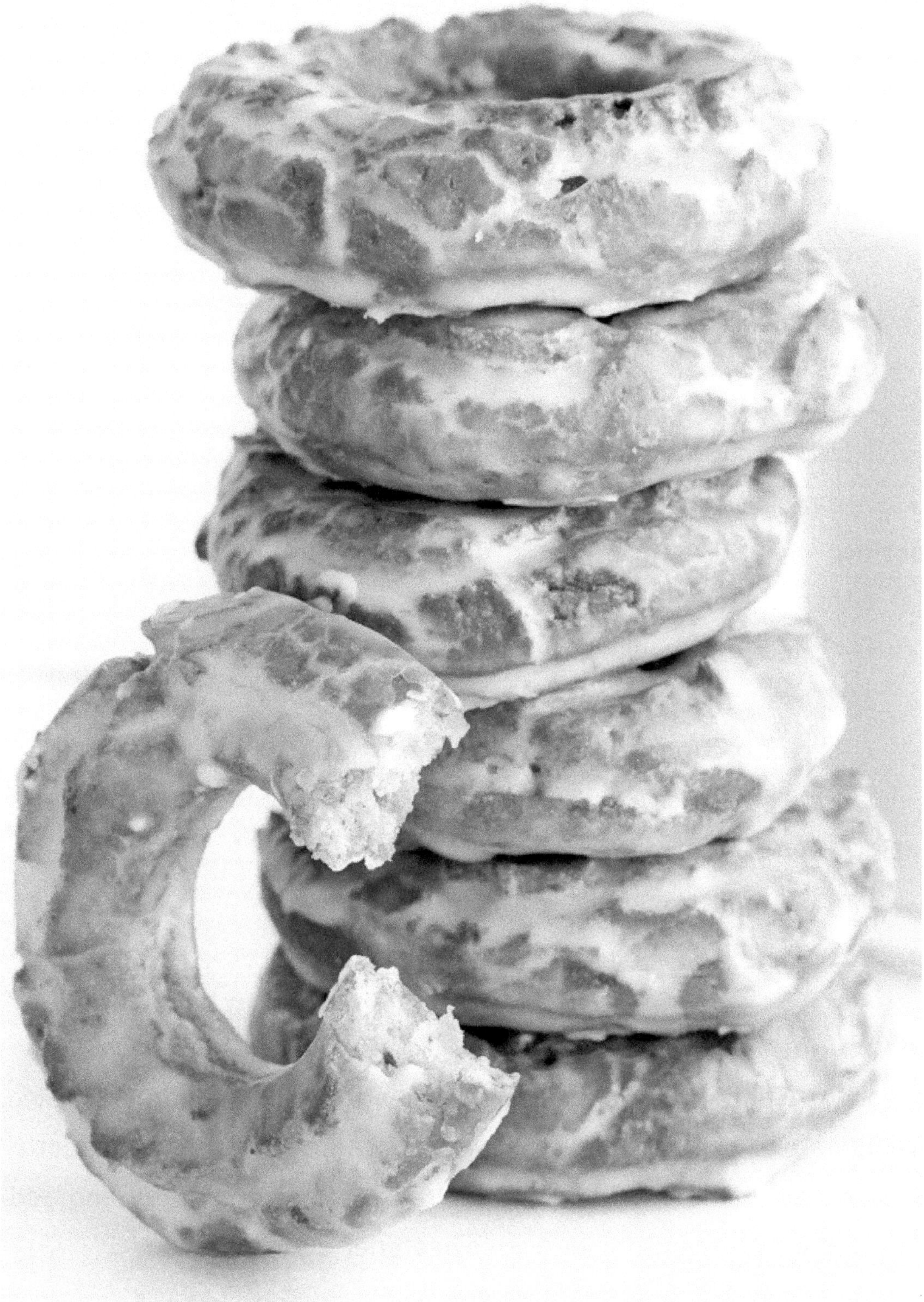

14 Nut-Free Chaffles

(Ready in about 30 minutes | Serving 3 | Difficulty: Easy)

Per serving: Kcal 195, Fat: 15.1g, Net Carbs: 31.5g, Protein: 8.5g

Ingredients

Batter

- 1/2 cup shredded cheese mozzarella
- 1/4 tsp of vanilla extract
- 2 tbsp of SunButter
- 2 tbsp of fruit sweetener
- 1 egg
- 2 tsp of cinnamon
- 1 tbsp of coconut flour
- ⅛ tsp of baking powder

Frosting

- 1 tbsp of cream cheese
- 1/4 cup of fruit sweetener
- 3/4 tbsp of butter, melted
- 1 tbsp of coconut milk unsweetened
- 1/4 tsp of vanilla extract

Coating

- 1 tsp of fruit sweetener
- 1 tsp of cinnamon

Instructions

Preheat the waffle iron. Mix batter ingredients in a bowl and place aside. Mix frosting ingredients except for coconut milk in a bowl and whisk until smooth. Add coconut milk and mix again. Place aside. Coat iron with cooking spray and add batter. Cook for around 4 minutes. Sprinkle with sweetener and cinnamon.

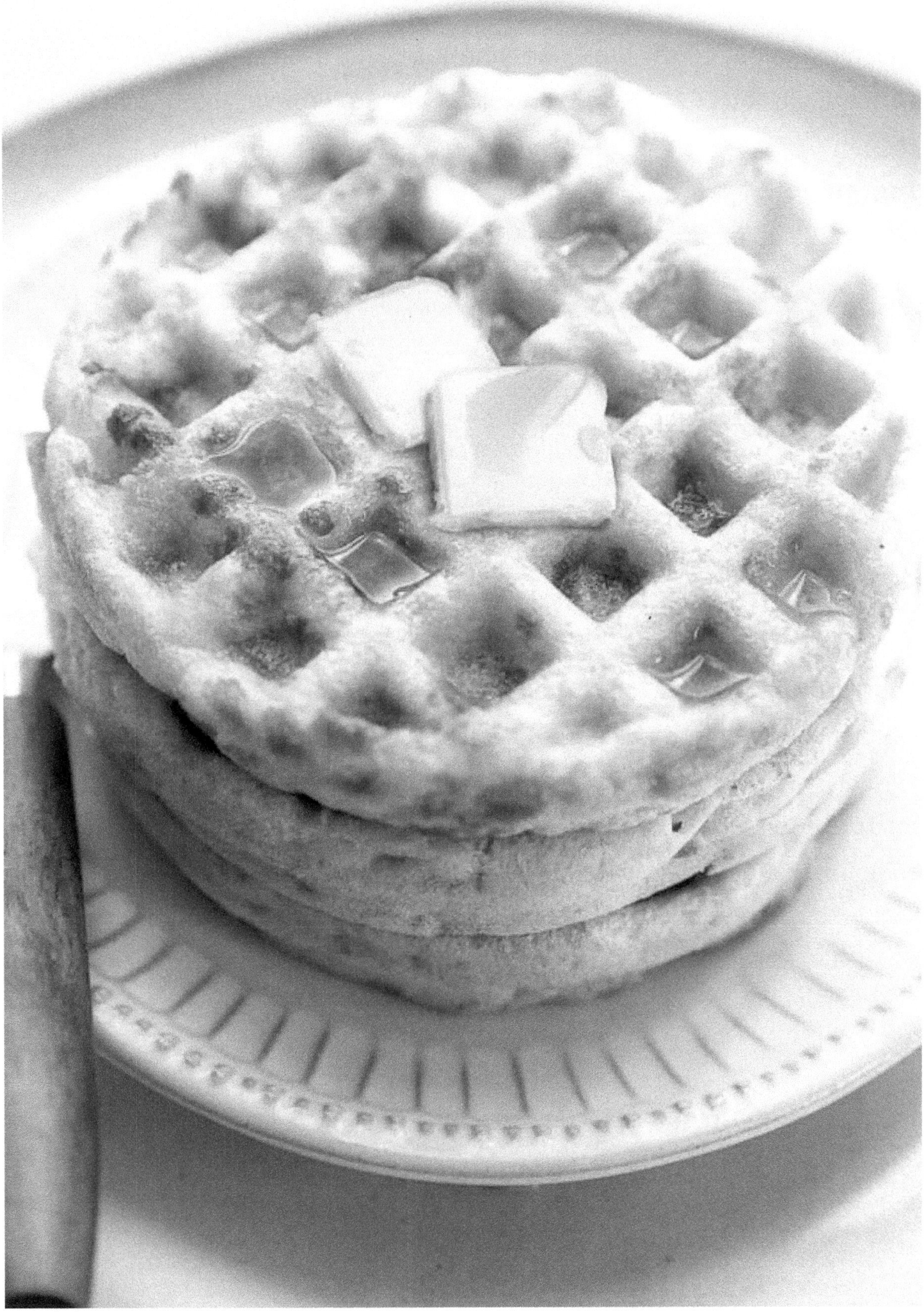

15 Chicken Chaffle

(Ready in about 19 minutes | Serving 2 | Difficulty: Easy)

Per serving: Kcal 675, Fat: 52g, Net Carbs: 8g, Protein: 44g

Ingredients

- 1/4 cup of almond flour
- 1/4 cup crumbled feta cheese
- 2 eggs
- 1 tsp of baking powder
- 1/2 cup shredded chicken
- 1/4 cup of Hot Sauce
- 1/4 cup shredded mozzarella cheese
- 3/4 cup shredded cheddar cheese
- 1/4 cup diced celery

Instructions

Mix almond flour and baking powder in a bowl. Preheat iron and spray using cooking spray. Beat eggs in a bowl and add hot sauce. Combine thoroughly and pour flour mixture. Combine and add grated cheeses. Fold in chicken. Pour in the maker and cook for around 4 minutes. Top with celery and feta.

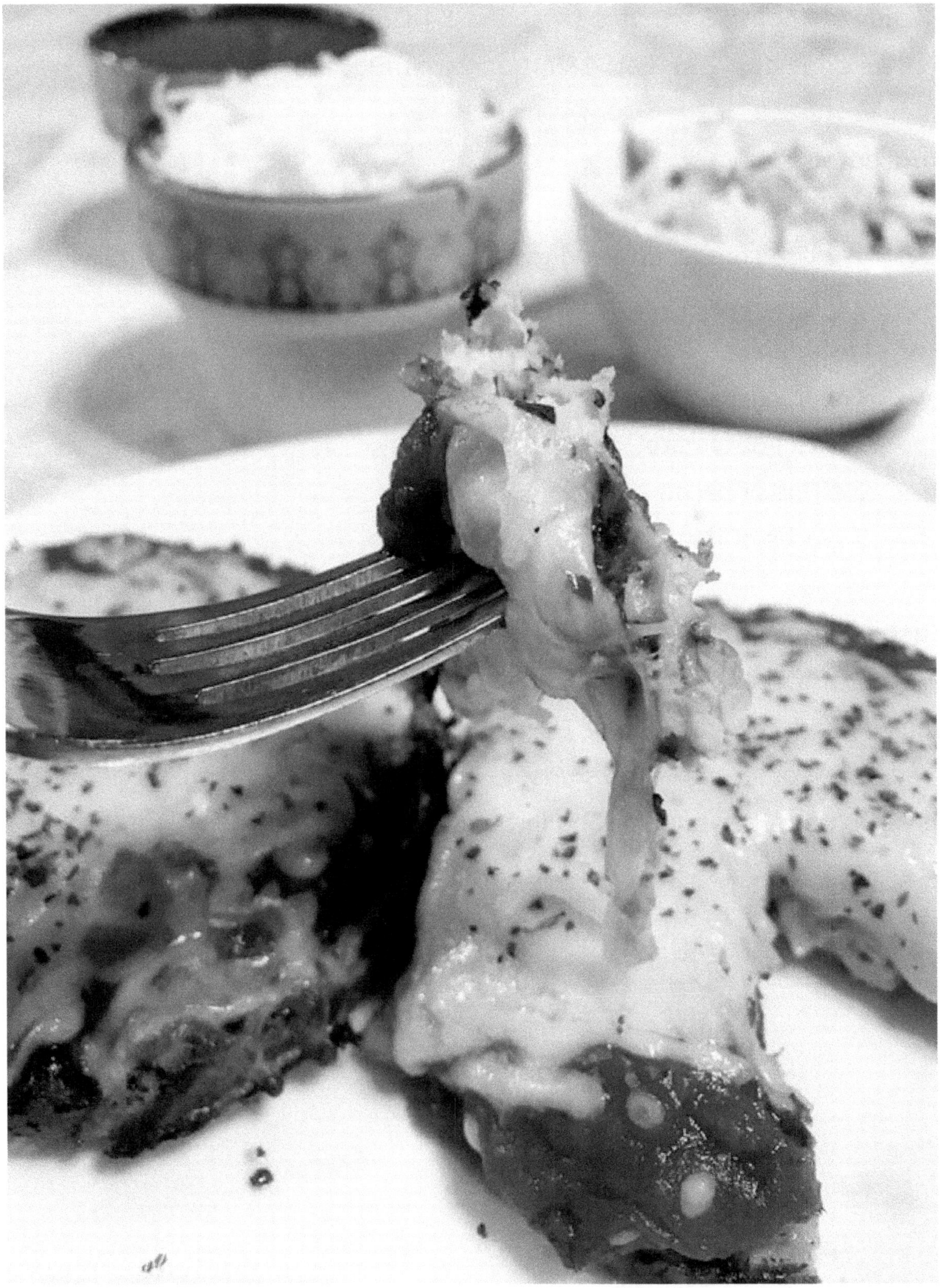

16 Chaffle Sandwich

(Ready in about 13 minutes | Serving 1 | Difficulty: Easy)

Per serving: Kcal 238, Fat: 18g, Net Carbs: 2g, Protein: 17g

Ingredients

For chaffles

- 1/2 cup shredded Cheddar cheese
- 1 egg

For sandwich

- 1 tbsp of mayonnaise
- 2 slices of tomato
- 2 strips of bacon
- 3 pieces of lettuce

Instructions

Preheat the maker and mix cheese and egg in a bowl. Pour batter into the maker and cook for around 4 minutes. Do it in 2 batches. Cook bacon in pan paced on the moderate flame until it gets crispy. Drain using paper towels and form a sandwich using tomato, mayonnaise and lettuce.

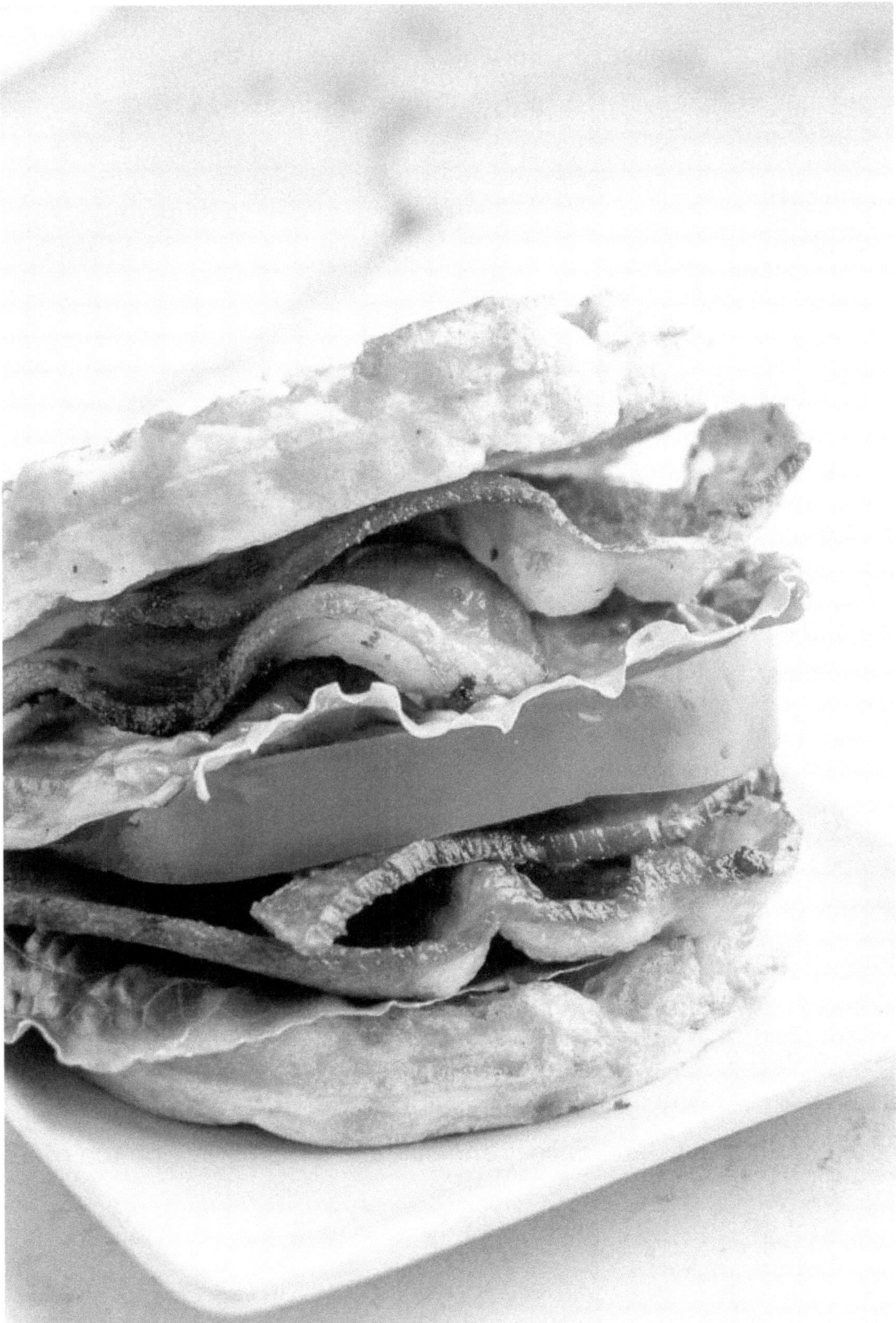

17 Sausage Gravy Chaffle

(Ready in about 15 minutes | Serving 2 | Difficulty: Easy)

Per serving: Kcal 212, Fat: 17g, Net Carbs: 3g, Protein: 11g

Ingredients

For Chaffle

- 1/2 cup grated mozzarella cheese
- 1 egg
- 1 tsp of coconut flour
- 1/4 tsp of baking powder
- 1 tsp of water
- Salt

For Gravy

- 3 tbsp of chicken broth
- 1/4 cup browned breakfast sausage
- 2 tbsp of whipping cream
- dash of garlic powder
- 2 tsp softened cream cheese
- pepper

Instructions

Preheat the maker and coat using cooking spray. Add all ingredients to a bowl and mix. Pour half amount to mixture into the maker and cook for around 4 minutes. Repeat with the remaining batter and enjoy. Prepare breakfast sausage and add in the pan with remaining ingredients and boil. Reduce flame and cook for around 7 minutes to thicken it. Add pepper and salt and spoon gravy on top of chaffles.

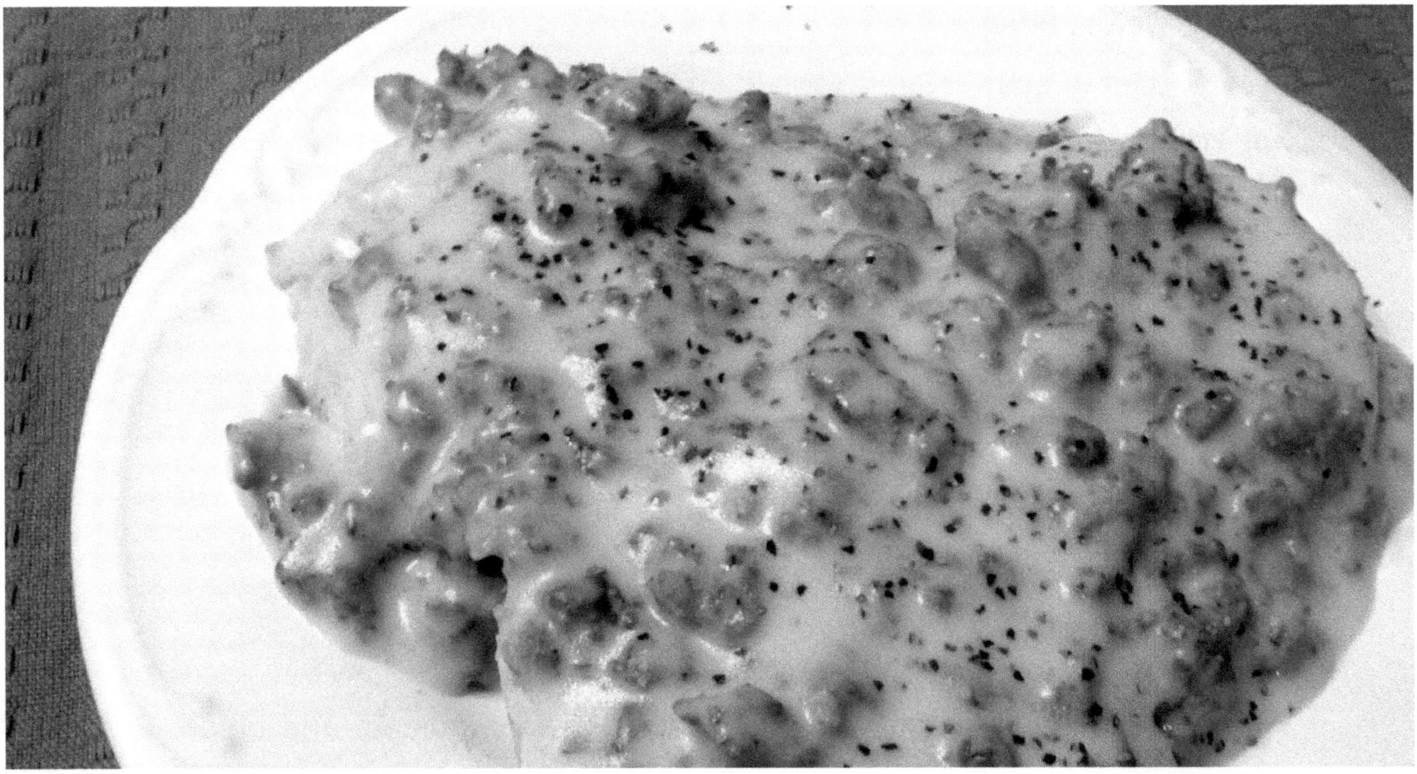

18 Eggs Benedict

(Ready in about 30 minutes | Serving 2 | Difficulty: Easy)

Per serving: Kcal 844, Fat: 78g, Net Carbs: 5g, Protein: 32g

Ingredients

For Chaffles

- 1/2 cup of mozzarella cheese
- 2 tbsp of almond flour
- 2 whites of eggs
- 1 tbsp of sour cream

For Hollandaise

- 2 tbsp of lemon juice
- 4 yolks of eggs
- 1/2 cup of salted butter

For Eggs

- 1 tbsp of white vinegar
- 3 ounces of deli ham
- 2 eggs

Instructions

Whisk eggs in a bowl and with the rest of the ingredients and blend. Preheat the waffle maker. Spray using cooking spray and add half the mixture. Cook for around 7 minutes. Make hollandaise sauce by forming a double broiler. Boil water and warm butter in the microwave. Add egg to bowl of the boiler. Boil and add hot butter while the pot is carried to a boil. Cook until egg thickens and take out of the bowl. Drizzle lemon juice and place aside. Warm chaffle using toaster and top with ham slices, 2 tbsp hollandaise sauce and one egg.

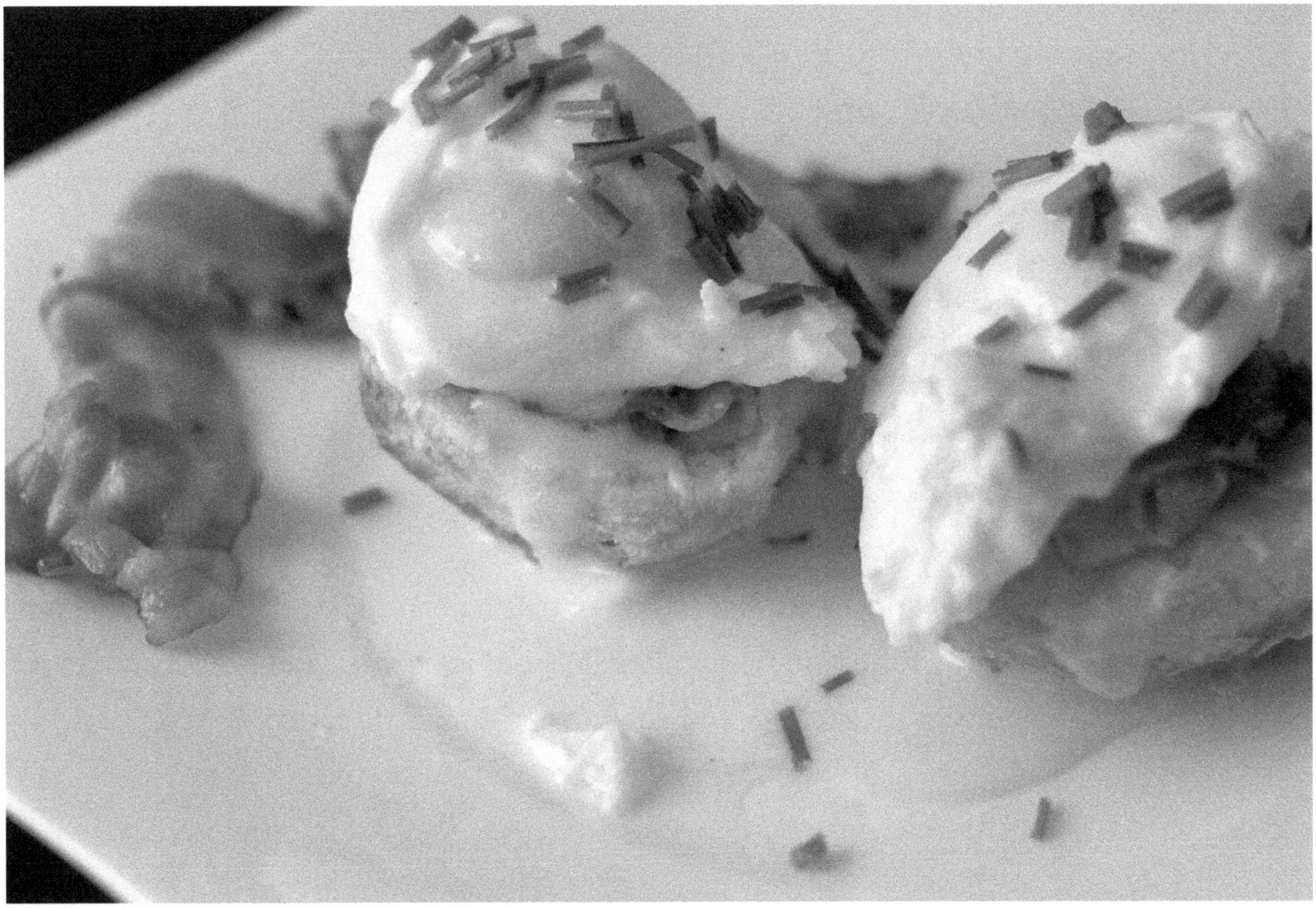

19 Garlic Chaffle

(Ready in about 10 minutes | Serving 8 | Difficulty: Easy)

Per serving: Kcal 74, Fat: 6.5g, Net Carbs: 0.9g, Protein: 3.4g

Ingredients

- 1 egg
- 2 tbsp of almond flour
- 1/2 cup grated mozzarella cheese
- 1/2tsp of garlic powder
- 1/2tsp of salt
- 1/2tsp of oregano

Topping

- 1/2tsp of garlic powder
- 2 tbsp softened butter
- 1/4 cup grated mozzarella cheese

Instructions

Preheat the maker and oil it. Mix ingredients except topping ingredients. Pour into the maker and cook for around 5 minutes. Mix garlic powder and butter and pour over waffle. Sprinkle with mozzarella and cook for around 3 minutes.

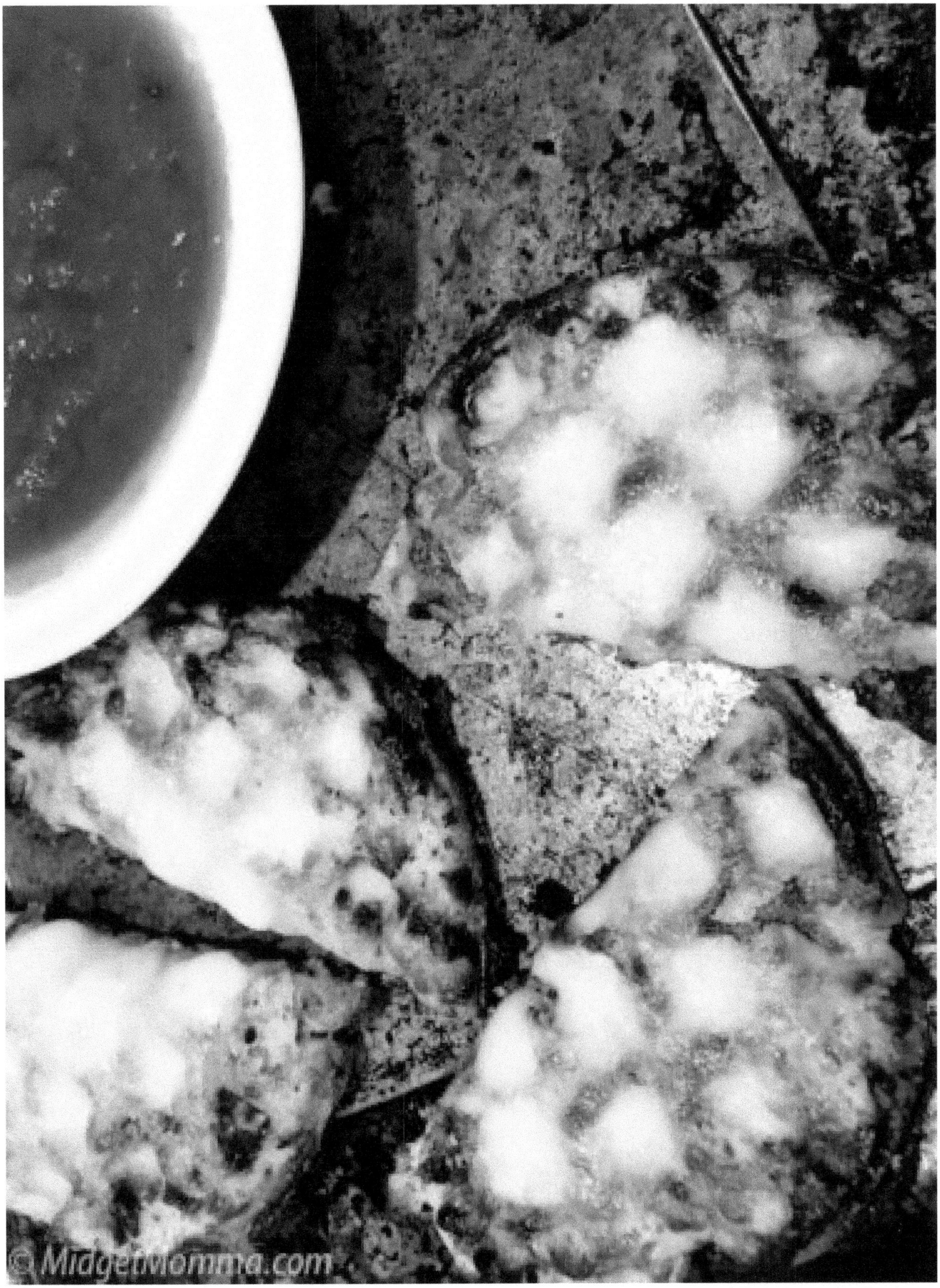
© MidgetMomma.com

20 Taco Chaffle

(Ready in about 13 minutes | Serving 1 | Difficulty: Easy)

Per serving: Kcal 258, Fat: 19g, Net Carbs: 4g, Protein: 18g

Ingredients

- 1/4 cup shredded jack cheese
- 1 white of egg
- 1/4 cup shredded cheddar cheese
- 1 tsp of coconut flour
- 3/4 tsp of water
- 1/4 tsp of baking powder
- pinch of salt
- 1/8 tsp of chili powder

Instructions

Preheat the maker and oil it. Combine everything in a bowl and spoon half amount of mixture in the maker. Cook for around 4 minutes. Remove the chaffle shell and place it aside. Repeat with the remaining batter. Turn the pan and position shells of the chaffle among cups to make a shell of taco.

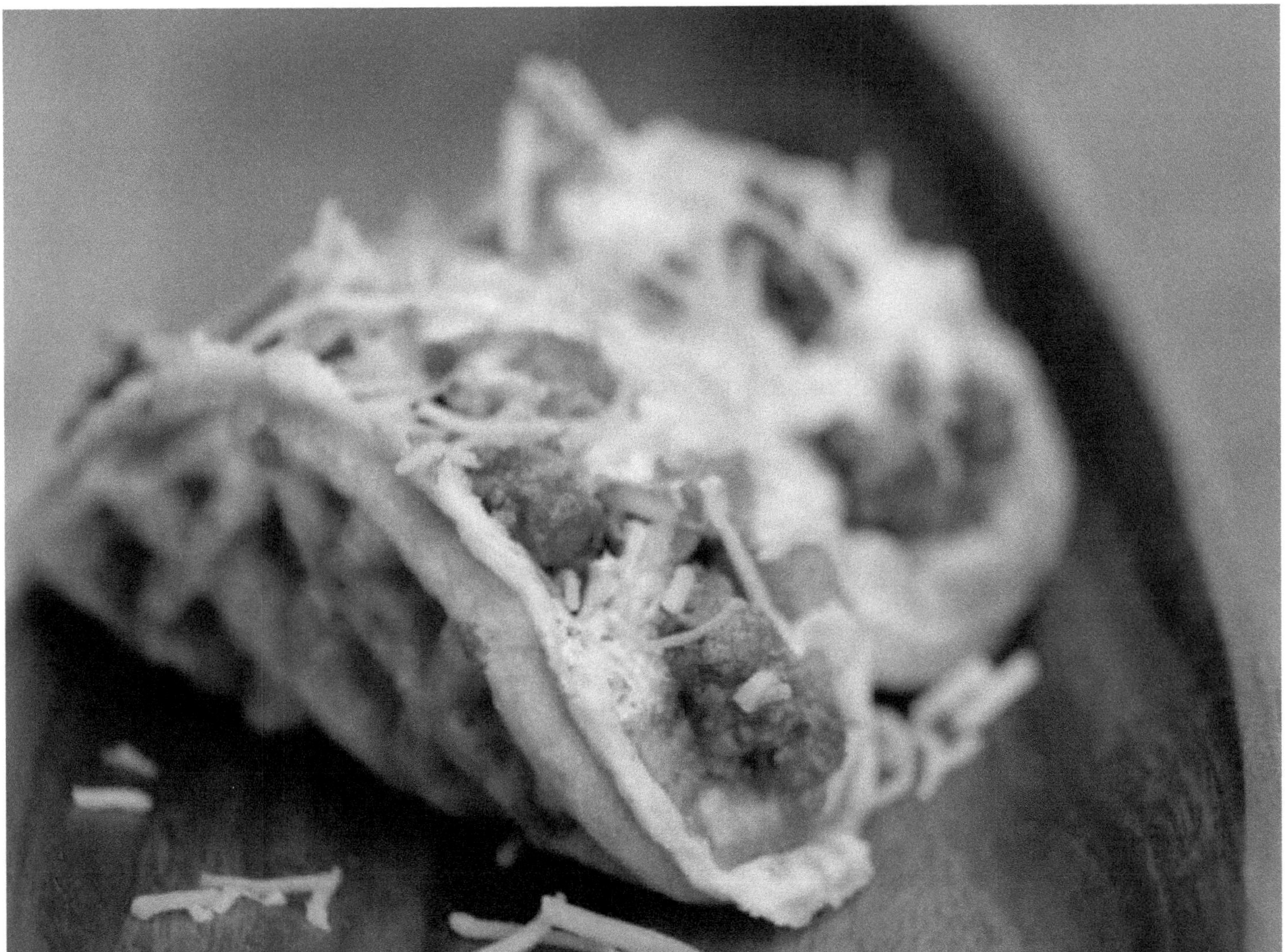
© LowCarbInspirations.com

21 Pizza Chaffle

(Ready in about 8 minutes | Serving 2 | Difficulty: Easy)

Per serving: Kcal 76, Fat: 4.3g, Net Carbs: 4.1g, Protein: 5.5g

Ingredients

- 1 egg
- Pinch of Italian seasoning
- 1/2 cup shredded mozzarella cheese
- 1 tbsp of pizza sauce

Instructions

Preheat the maker. Whisk eggs in a bowl and add seasonings. Mix shredded cheese in a bowl. Add half amount of mixture to the maker and cook for around 4 minutes. Repeat with the rest of the batter and with 1 tbsp pizza sauce and pepperoni.

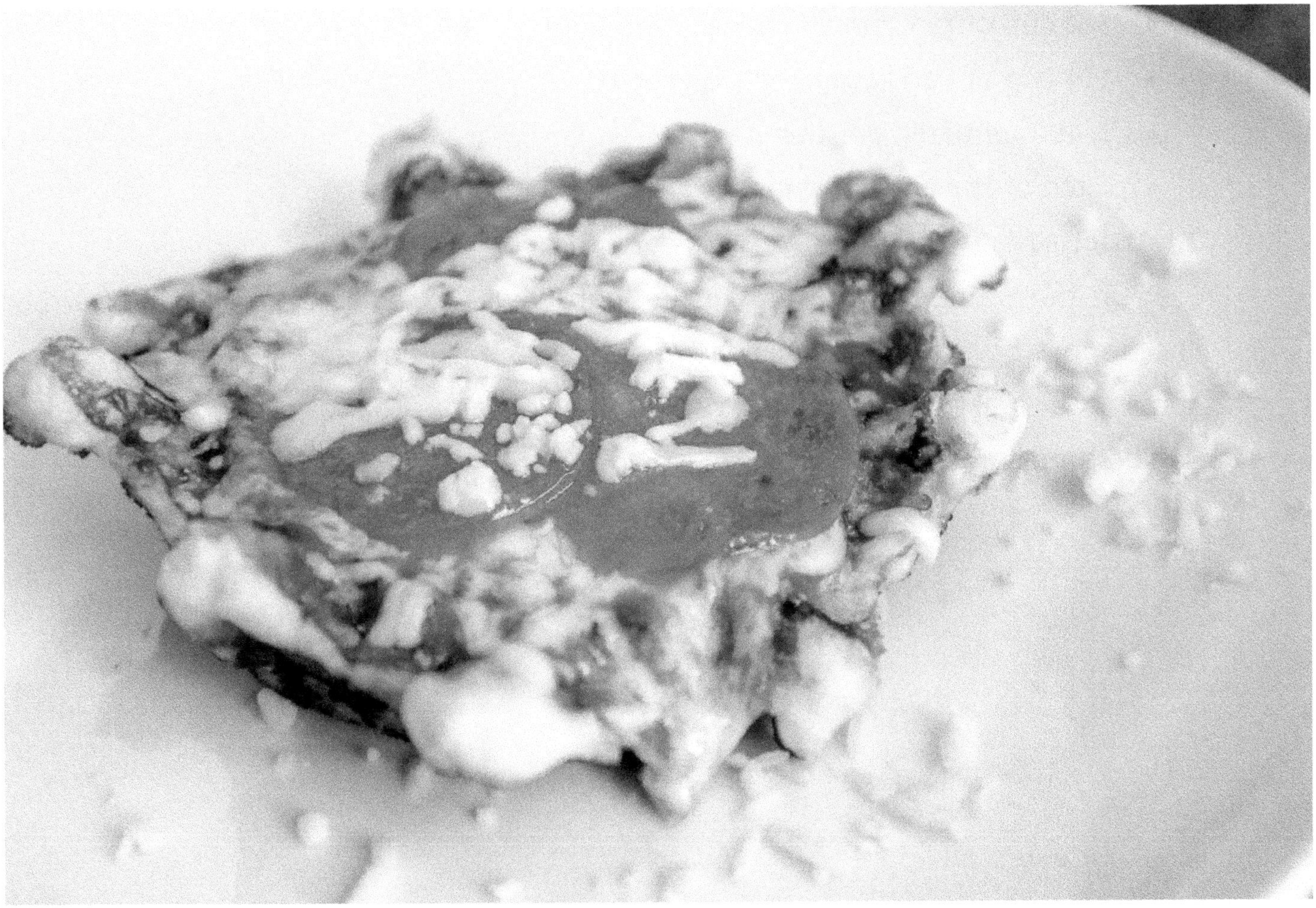

22 Parmesan Chaffles

(Ready in about 6 minutes | Serving 1 | Difficulty: Easy)

Per serving: Kcal 352, Fat: 24g, Net Carbs: 2g, Protein: 14g

Ingredients

- 1 beaten egg
- 1/2 cup of mozzarella cheese shredded
- 1/4 cup of Parmesan cheese grated
- 1/4tsp of garlic powder
- 1 tsp of Italian seasoning

Instructions

Preheat the waffle maker. Add all the ingredients except mozzarella and parmesan cheese in a bowl and mix. Mix the cheese in a bowl and spray waffle sung cooking spray. Pour half amount of mixture in the maker and cook for around 5 minutes. Top using parmesan and enjoy.

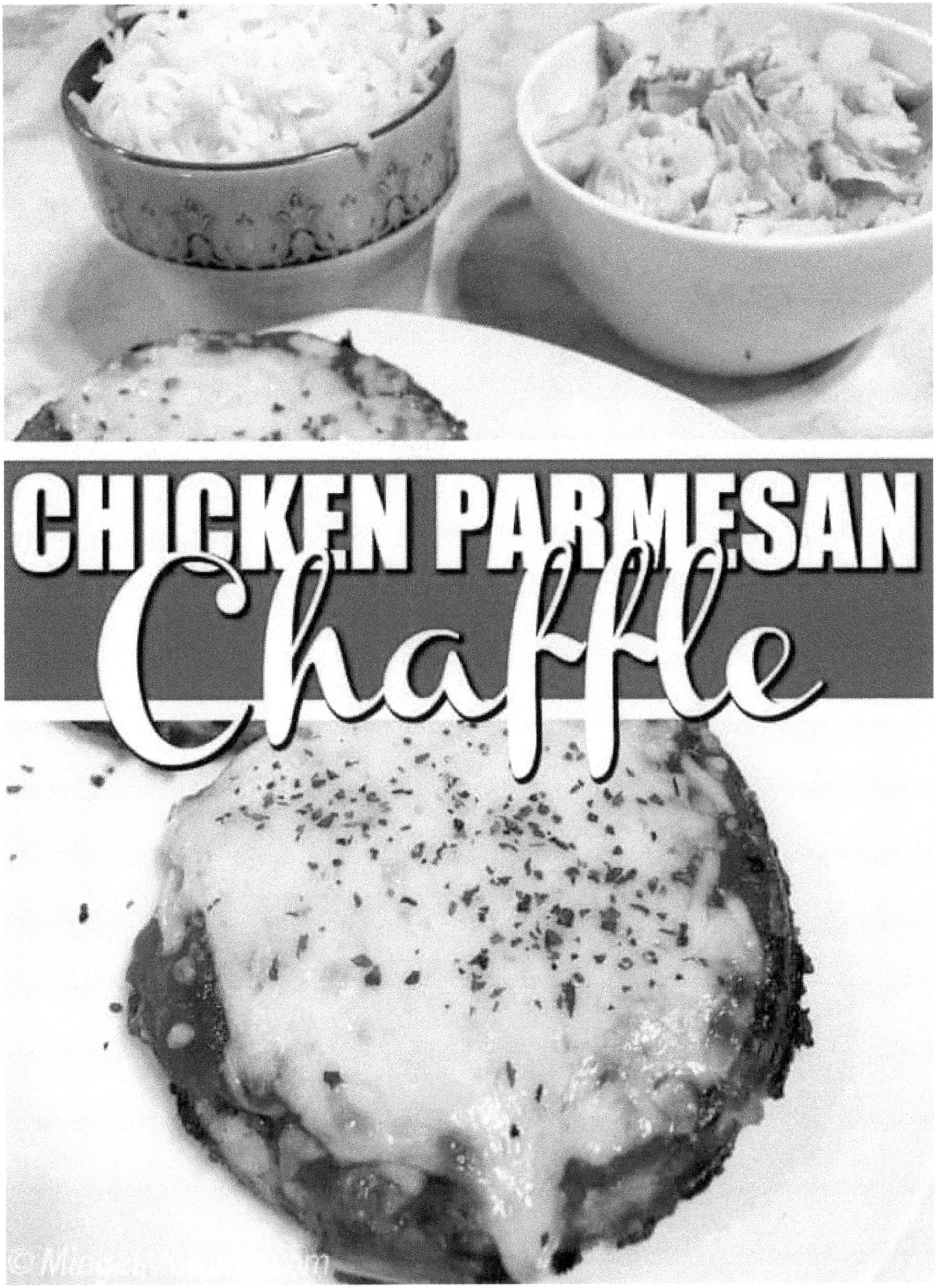
CHICKEN PARMESAN
Chaffle

23 Italian Chaffle

(Ready in about 6 minutes | Serving 1 | Difficulty: Easy)

Per serving: Kcal 352, Fat: 24g, Net Carbs: 2g, Protein: 14g

Ingredients

- 1 beaten egg
- 1/2 cup of mozzarella cheese shredded
- 1/4 cup of Parmesan cheese grated
- 1/4tsp of garlic powder
- 1 tsp of Italian seasoning

Instructions

Preheat the waffle maker. Add all the ingredients except mozzarella and parmesan cheese in a bowl and mix. Mix the cheese in a bowl and spray waffle sung cooking spray. Pour half amount of mixture in the maker and cook for around 5 minutes. Top using parmesan and add lettuce, cold cuts, tomato.

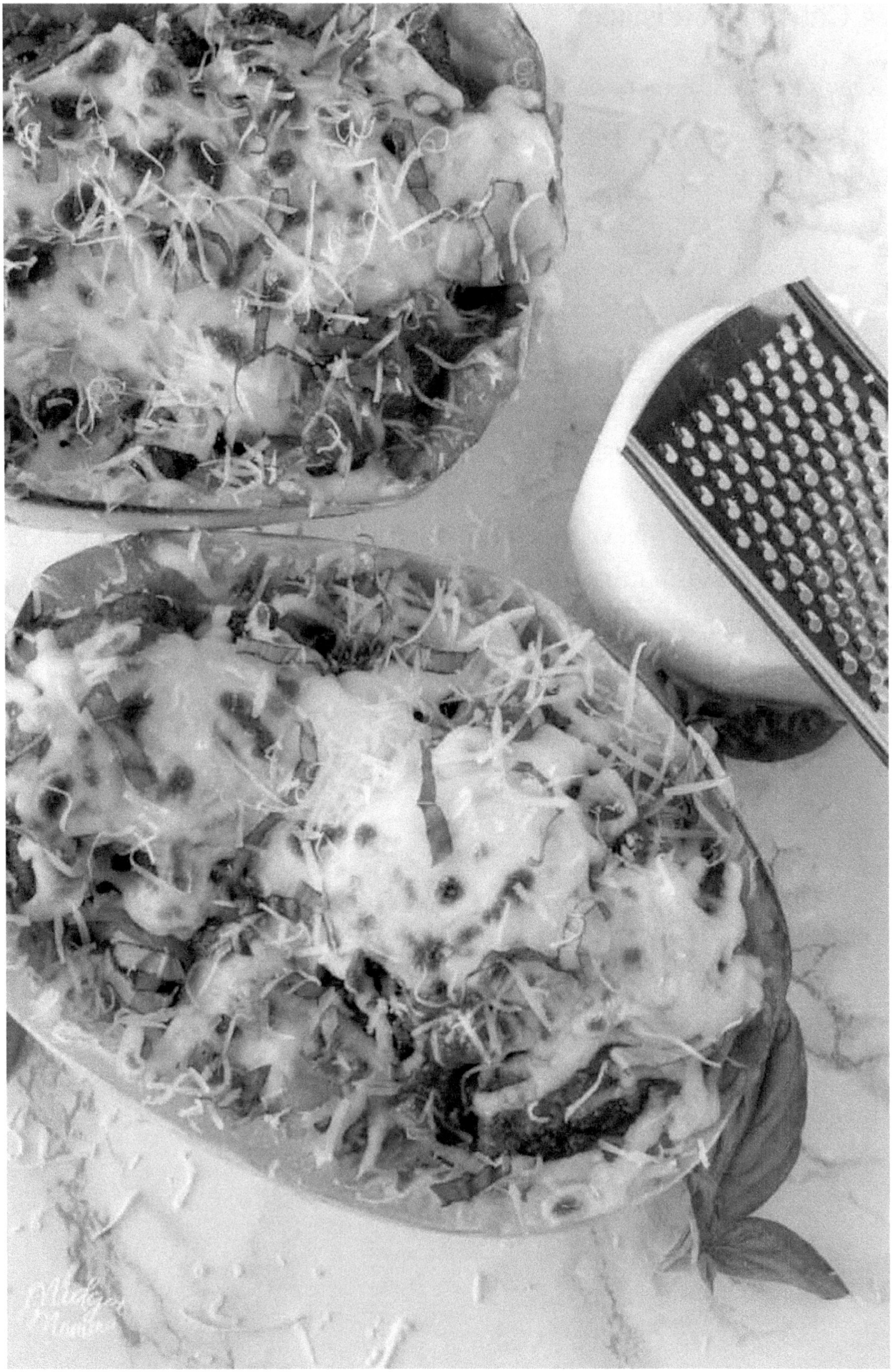

24 Chaffle Breadsticks

(Ready in about 6 minutes | Serving 1 | Difficulty: Easy)

Per serving: Kcal 352, Fat: 24g, Net Carbs: 2g, Protein: 14g

Ingredients

- 1 beaten egg
- 1/2 cup of mozzarella cheese shredded
- Marinara sauce
- 1/4 cup of Parmesan cheese grated
- 1/4tsp of garlic powder
- 1 tsp of Italian seasoning

Instructions

Preheat the waffle maker. Add all the ingredients except mozzarella and parmesan cheese in a bowl and mix. Mix the cheese in a bowl and spray waffle sung cooking spray. Pour half amount of mixture in the maker and cook for around 5 minutes. Top using parmesan and dice into 4 sticks and enjoy with Marinara Sauce.

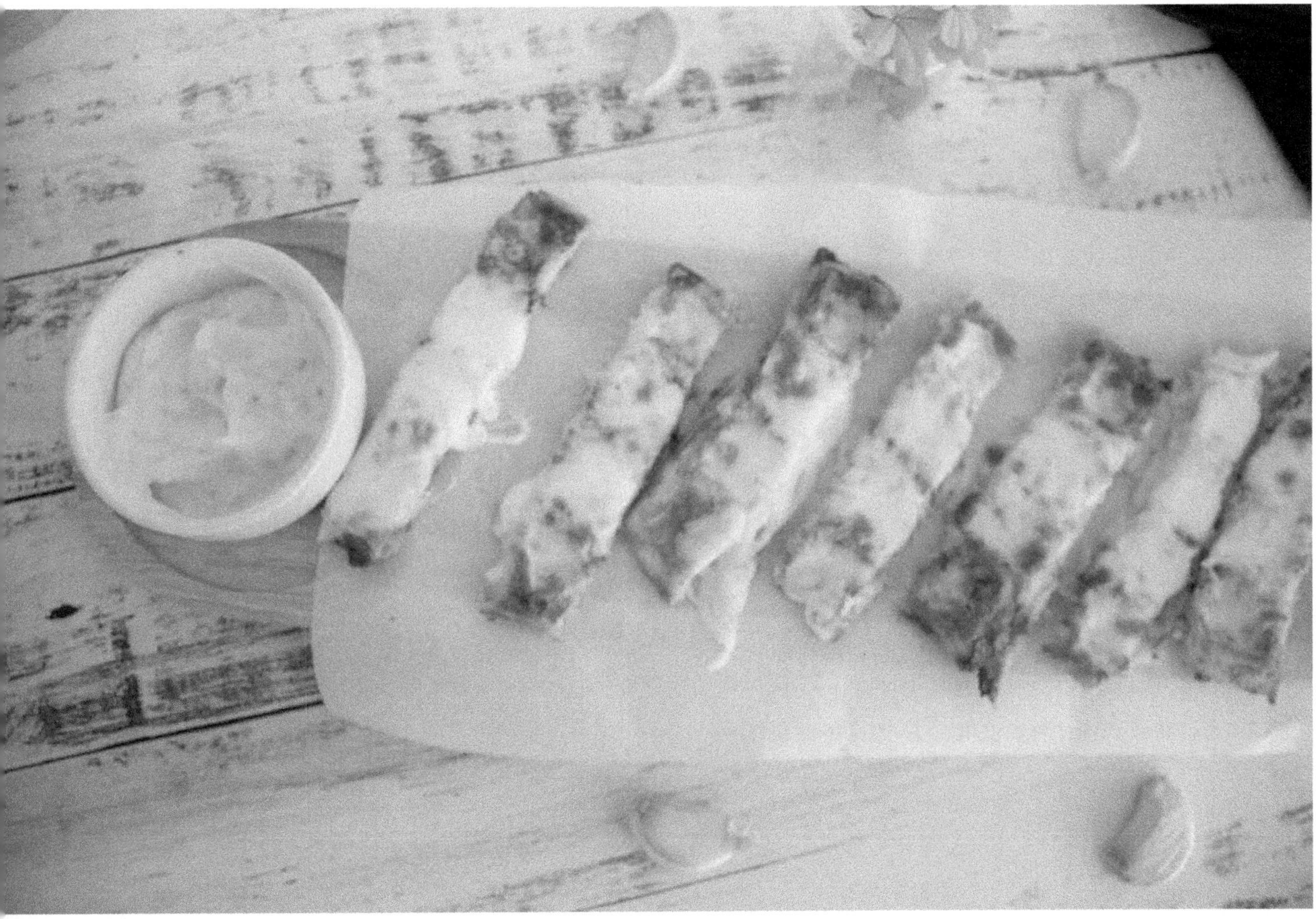

25 Chaffle Bruschetta

(Ready in about 6 minutes | Serving 1 | Difficulty: Easy)

Per serving: Kcal 352, Fat: 24g, Net Carbs: 2g, Protein: 14g

Ingredients

- 1 beaten egg
- 1/2 cup of mozzarella cheese shredded
- 1/4 cup of Parmesan cheese grated
- Basil
- Olive oil
- 1/4tsp of garlic powder
- 1 tsp of Italian seasoning

Instructions

Preheat the waffle maker. Add all the ingredients except mozzarella and parmesan cheese in a bowl and mix. Mix the cheese in a bowl and spray waffle sung cooking spray. Pour half amount of mixture in the maker and cook for around 5 minutes. Top using parmesan and mix 4 chopped cherry tomatoes, ½ tsp chopped fresh basil, drop of olive oil and salt. Add on chaffle.

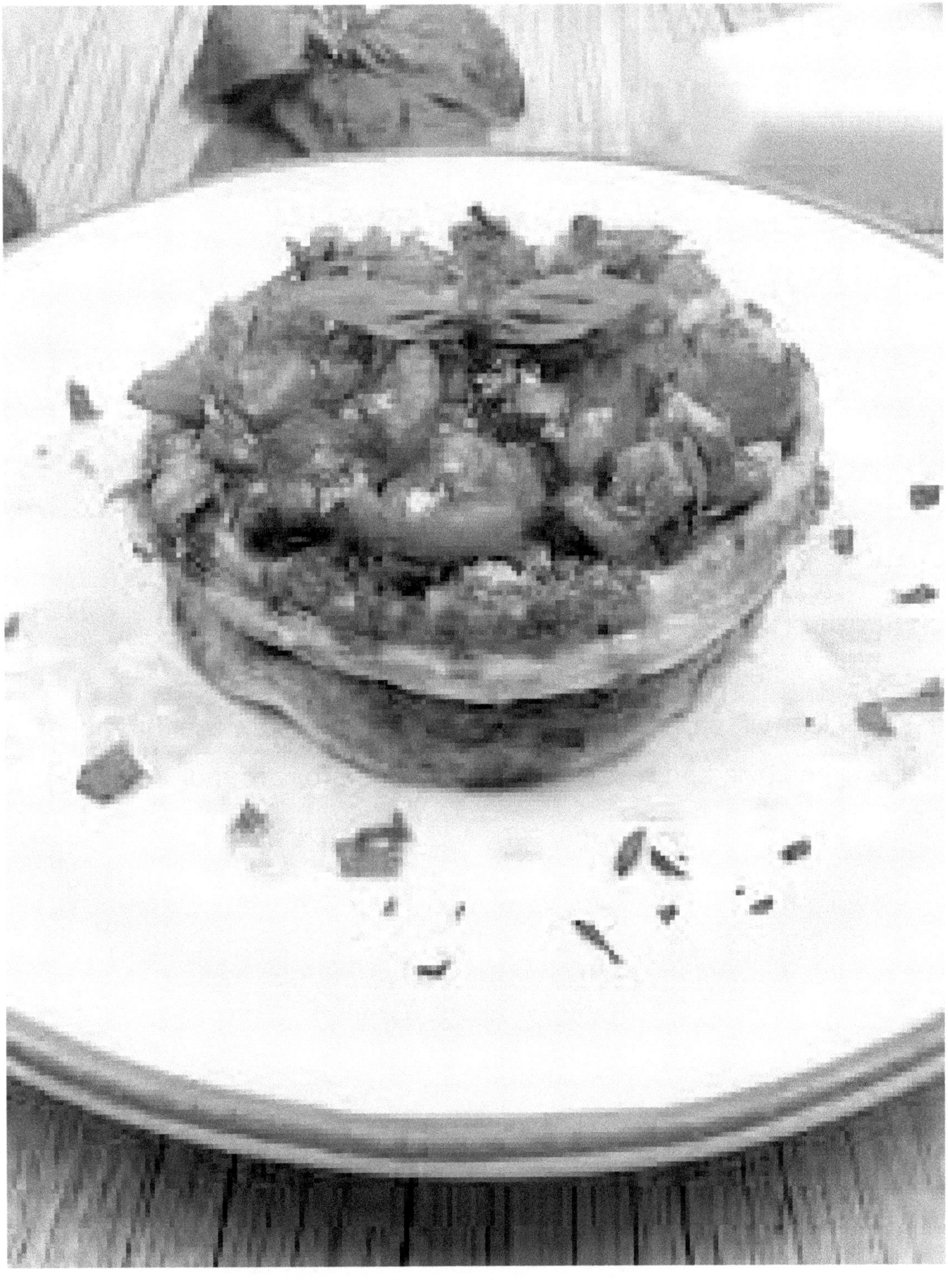

26 Cauliflower Chaffles

(Ready in about 9 minutes | Serving 2 | Difficulty: Easy)

Per serving: Kcal 246, Fat: 16g, Net Carbs: 7g, Protein: 20g

Ingredients

- 1/4 tsp of Garlic Powder
- 1 cup of riced cauliflower
- 1/4 tsp of Ground Black Pepper
- 1/4 tsp of Kosher Salt
- 1/2 tsp of Italian seasoning
- 1 Eggs
- 1/2 cup of mozzarella cheese shredded
- 1/2 cup of parmesan cheese shredded

Instructions

Blend all ingredients except the cauliflower mixture and parmesan cheese in a blender and sprinkle half parmesan in the maker. Pour mixture in maker and top with cauliflower mixture and rest of parmesan. Cook for around 5 minutes.

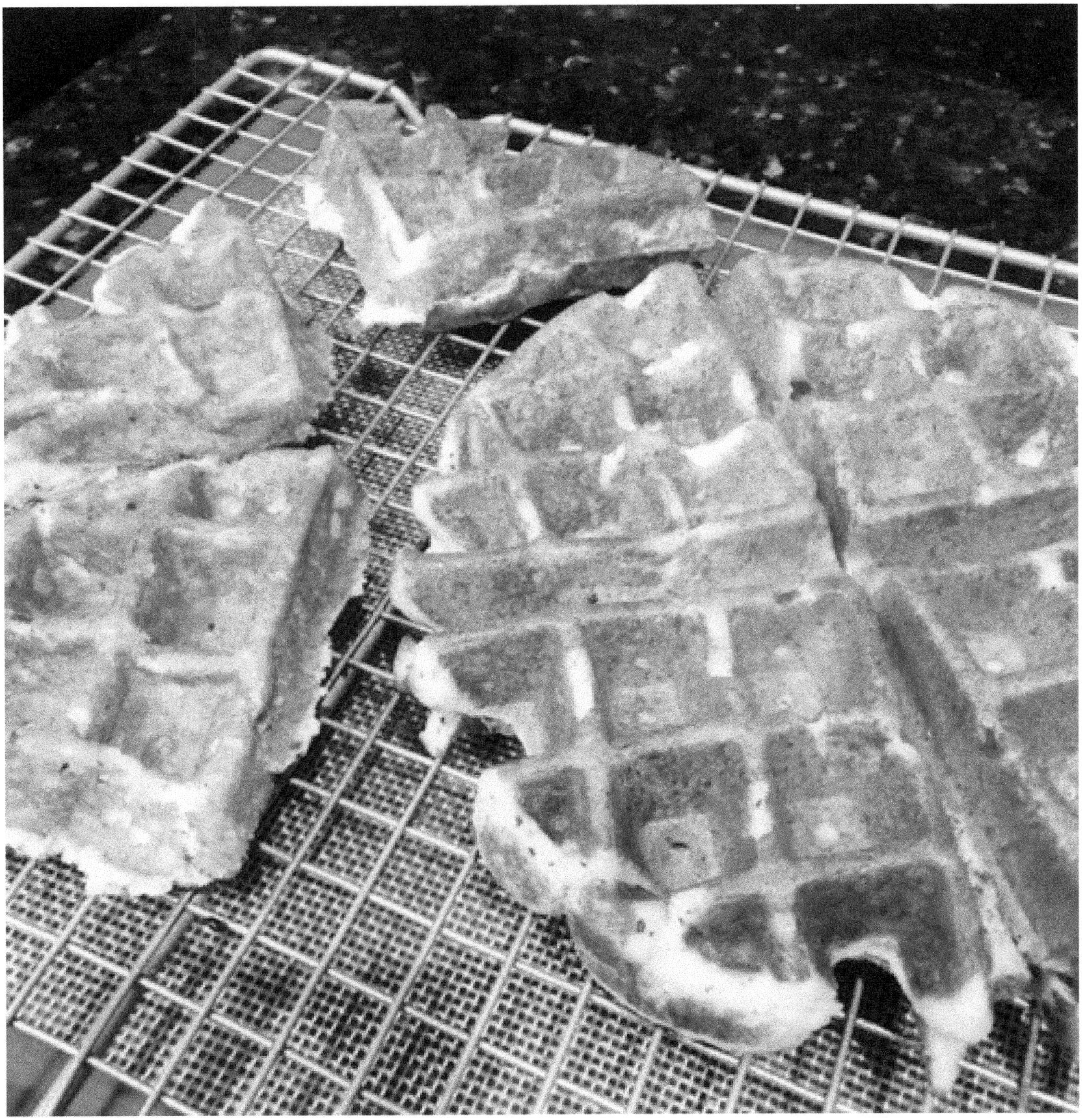

27 Zucchini Chaffles

(Ready in about 15 minutes | Serving 2 | Difficulty: Easy)

Per serving: Kcal 194, Fat: 13g, Net Carbs: 4g, Protein: 16g

Ingredients

- 1 beaten Egg
- 1/2 tsp Black Pepper Ground
- 1 cup grated Zucchini
- 1/2 cup of parmesan cheese shredded
- 1 tsp chopped Dried Basil
- 1/4 cup of mozzarella cheese shredded
- 3/4 tsp divided Kosher Salt

Instructions

Sprinkle 1/4 tsp salt on zucchini. Beat egg in a bowl and add mozzarella, zucchini, 1/2 tsp salt, basil and pepper. Sprinkle 2 tbsp parmesan on iron and spread a quarter of zucchini mixture on the maker. Top using 2 tbsp parmesan and cook for around 8 minutes. Repeat with the rest of the mixture.

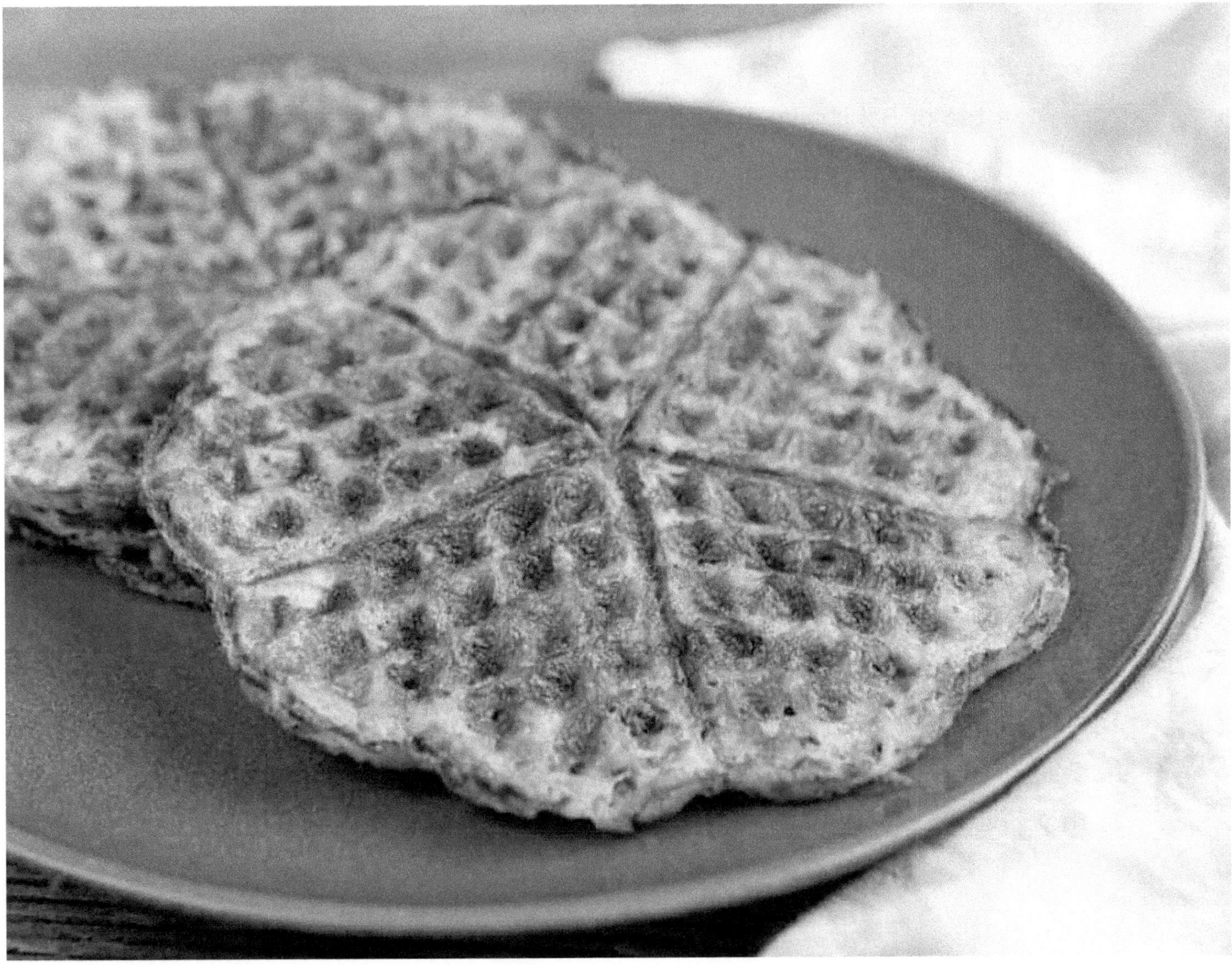

28 Peanut Chaffles

(Ready in about 6 minutes | Serving 2 | Difficulty: Easy)

Per serving: Kcal 264, Fat: 21.6g, Net Carbs: 7.25g, Protein: 9.45g

Ingredients

Chaffle

- 1 Egg
- 1/4 tsp of Baking Powder
- 1 tbsp of Unsweetened Cocoa
- 1 tbsp of Heavy Cream
- 1 tbsp of Powdered Sweetener
- 1/2 tsp of Vanilla Extract
- 1 tsp of Coconut Flour
- 1/2 tsp of Batter Flavor

Butter Filling

- 2 tsp of Powdered Sweetener
- 3 tbsp of Peanut Butter
- 2 tbsp of Heavy Cream

InstructionsPreheat the maker. Combine ingredients of chaffle in a bowl and pour half amount of mixture in maker. Cook for around 5 minutes. Repeat with the rest of the mixture. Blend butter ingredients and spread over chaffles.

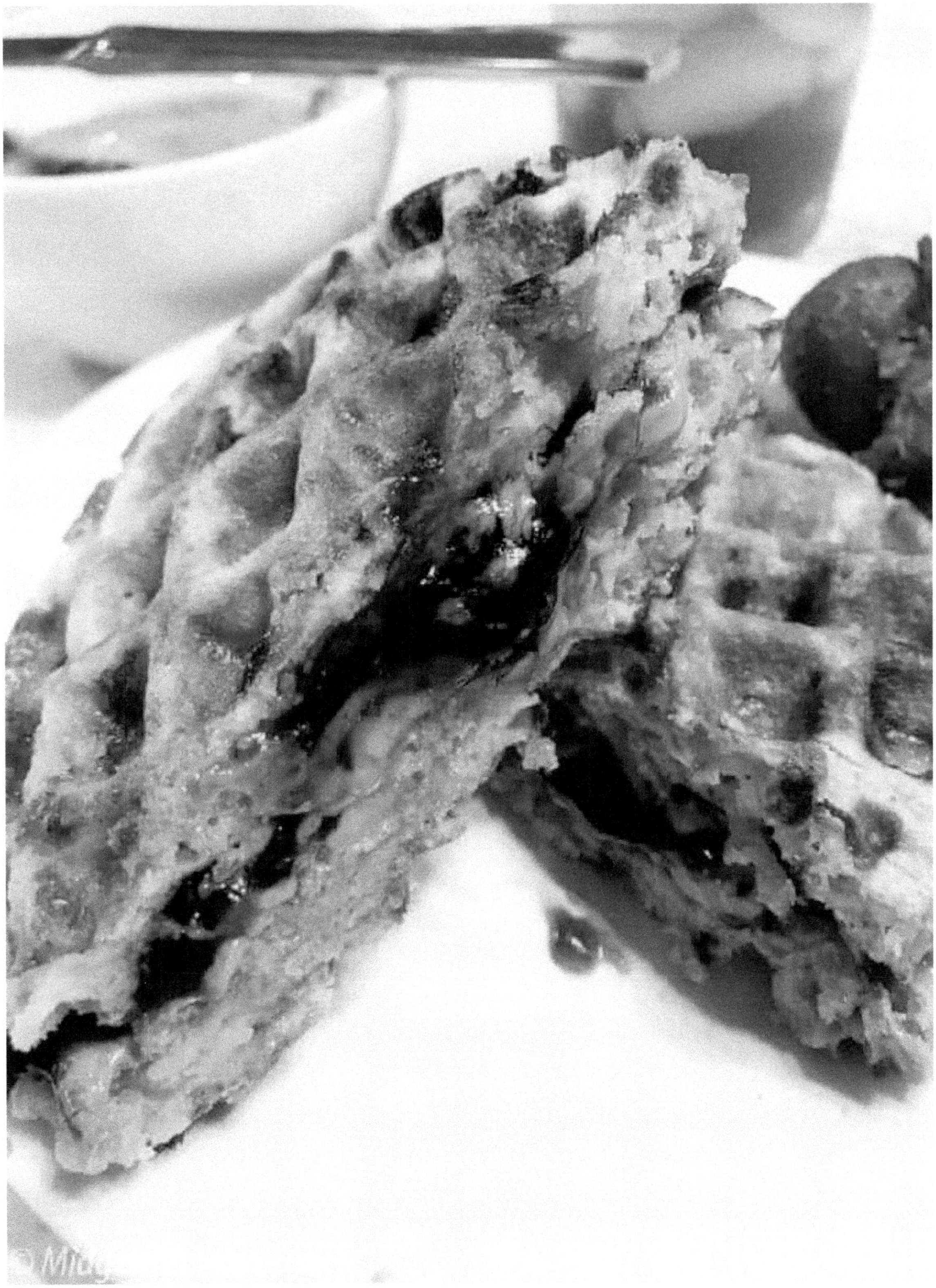

29 Easy Chaffle Recipe

(Ready in about 10 minutes | Serving 2| Difficulty: Easy)

Ingredients

Simple Chaffles

Per serving: Kcal 152, Fat: 8g, Net Carbs: 1g, Protein: 9g

- 1 Egg
- 1/2 Cup of Shredded Cheese Mozarella

Instructions

Add all ingredients to a bowl and whisk to combine. Coat waffle maker using cooking spray and pour half amount of batter into the maker. Cook for around 5 minutes and repeat with the rest of the batter.

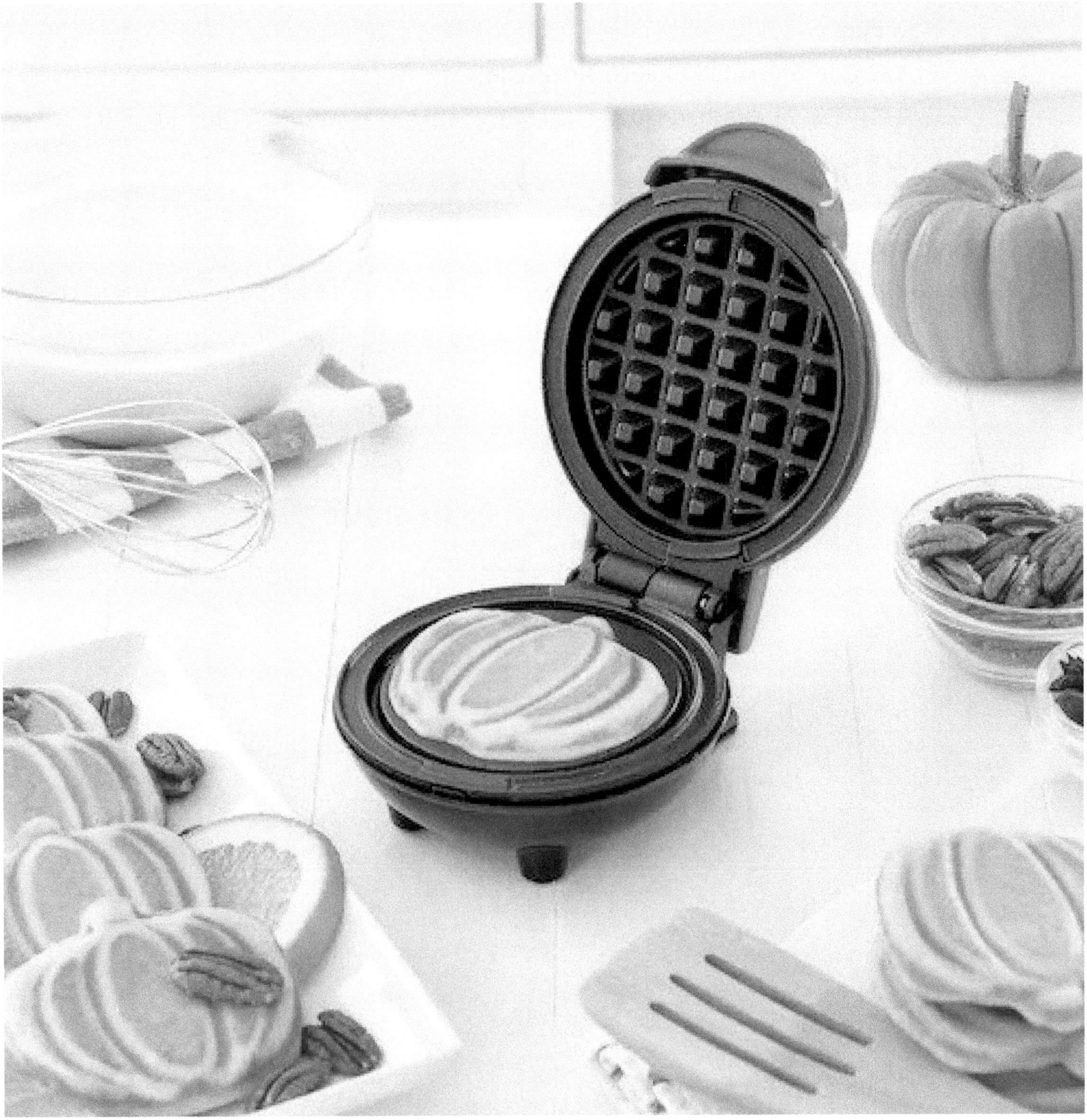

30 Savory Chaffles

Per serving: Kcal 215, Fat: 16.5g, Net Carbs: 2g, Protein: 12g

- 1 Egg
- 1/2 Cup Shredded Cheese Mozarella
- 1/16 Tsp of Xanthan Gum
- 1/4 Cup of Almond Flour

Instructions

Add all ingredients to a bowl and whisk to combine. Coat waffle maker using cooking spray and pour half amount of batter into the maker. Cook for around 5 minutes and repeat with the rest of the batter.

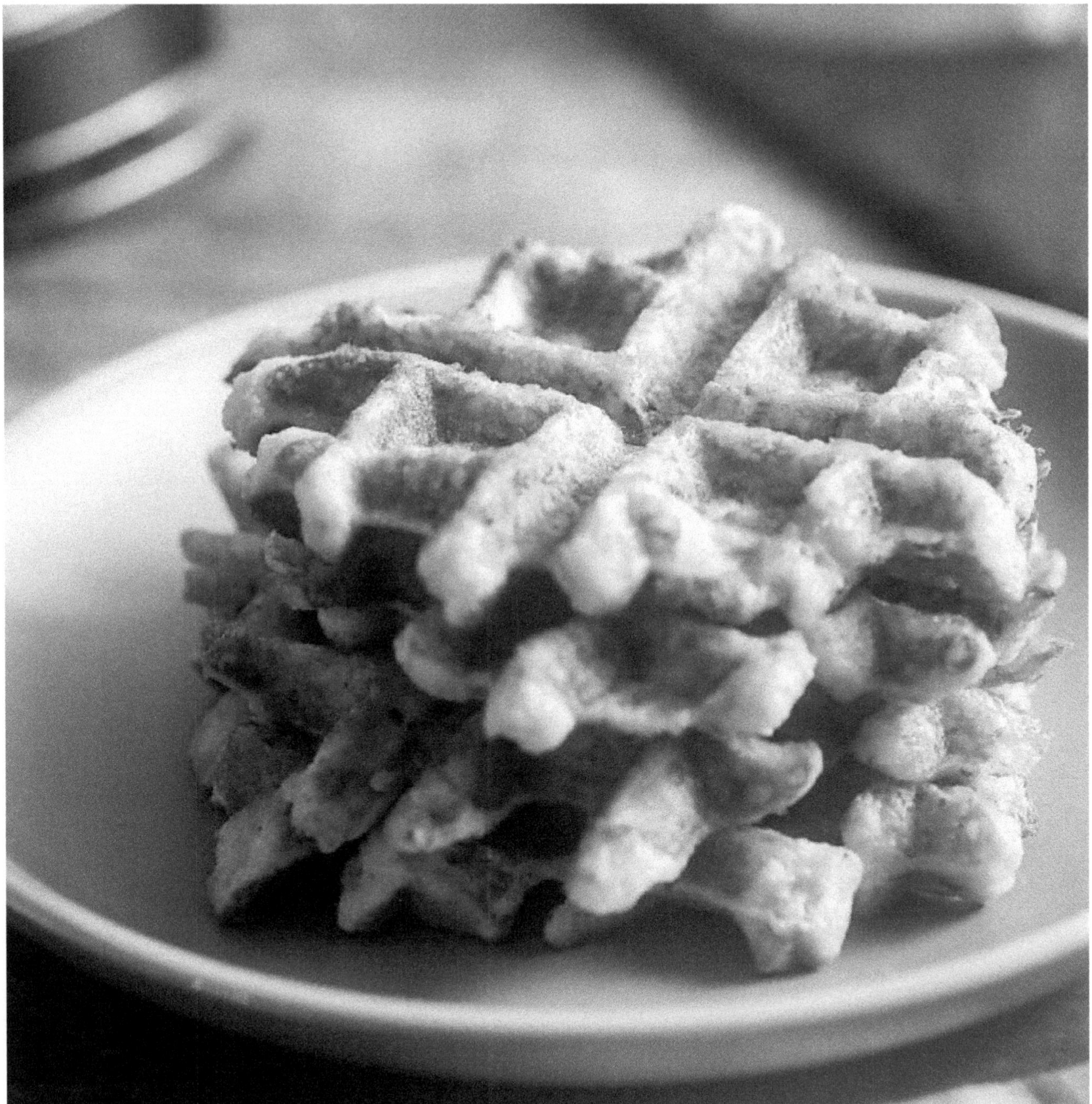

31 Sweet Chaffles

Per serving: Kcal 192, Fat: 15gg, Net Carbs: 1.55g, Protein: 15g

- 1 Egg
- 1/2 Cup of Shredded Cheese Mozzarella
- 1/4 Cup of Almond Flour
- 1/16 Tsp of Xanthan Gum
- 2 Tbsp of Confectioners Swerve

Instructions

Add all ingredients to a bowl and whisk to combine. Coat waffle maker using cooking spray and pour half amount of batter into the maker. Cook for around 5 minutes and repeat with the rest of the batter.

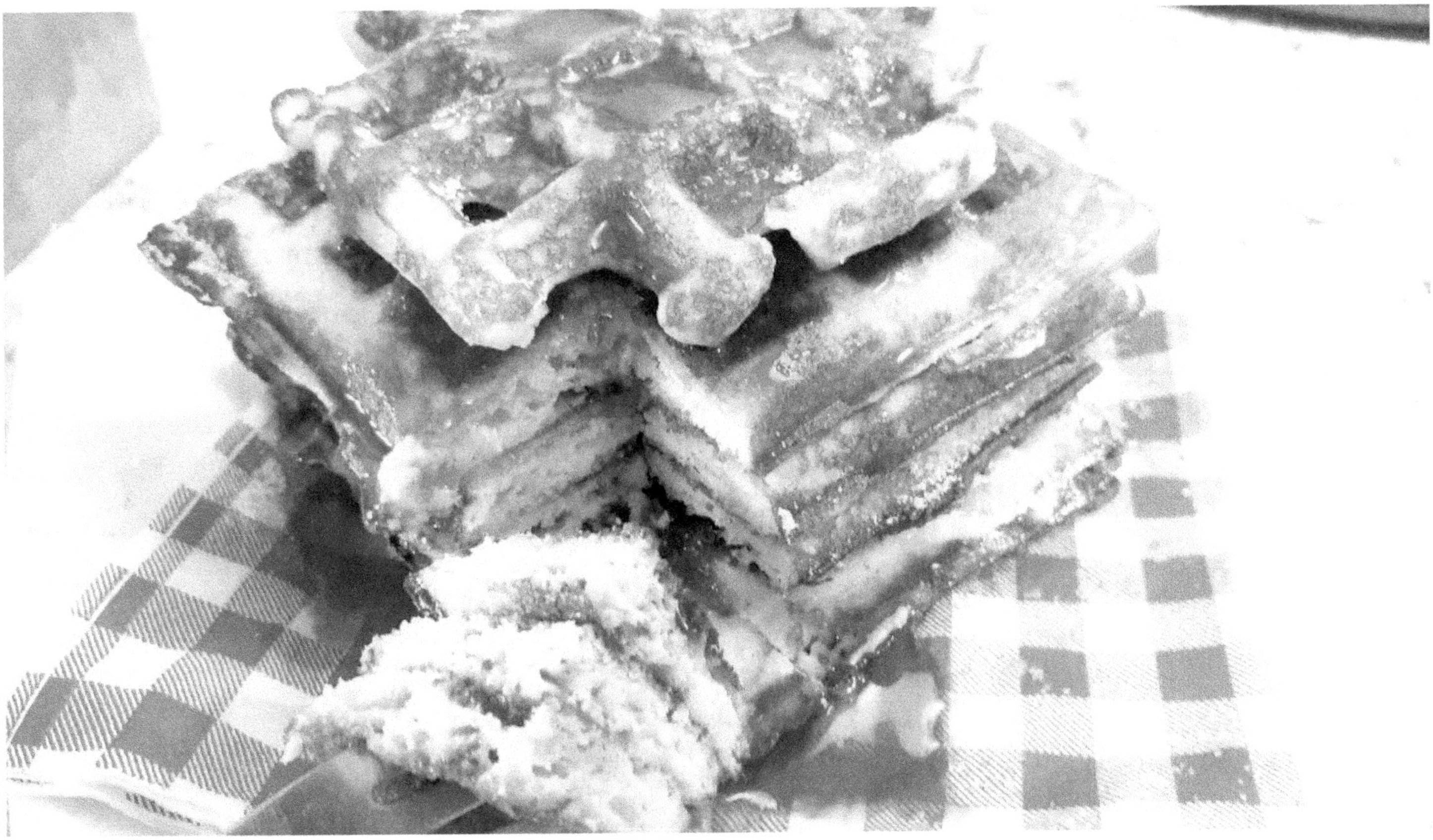

32 Tasty Chaffles

(Ready in about 13 minutes | Serving 2 | Difficulty: Easy)

Per serving: Kcal 116, Fat: 9.5gg, Net Carbs: 2.6g, Protein: 4.5g

Ingredients

- 1 oz softened cream cheese
- 1 tbsp of almond flour
- 1 tbsp of pumpkin puree
- 1 egg
- 1/2 tsp of pumpkin spice

Instructions

Whisk the cream cheese in a bowl. Whisk pumpkin puree and egg in a bowl. Add almond flour and pumpkin spice and mix. Preheat the iron and spray using oil. Pour half amount of mixture in the maker and cook for around 5 minutes. Repeat with the rest of the batter.

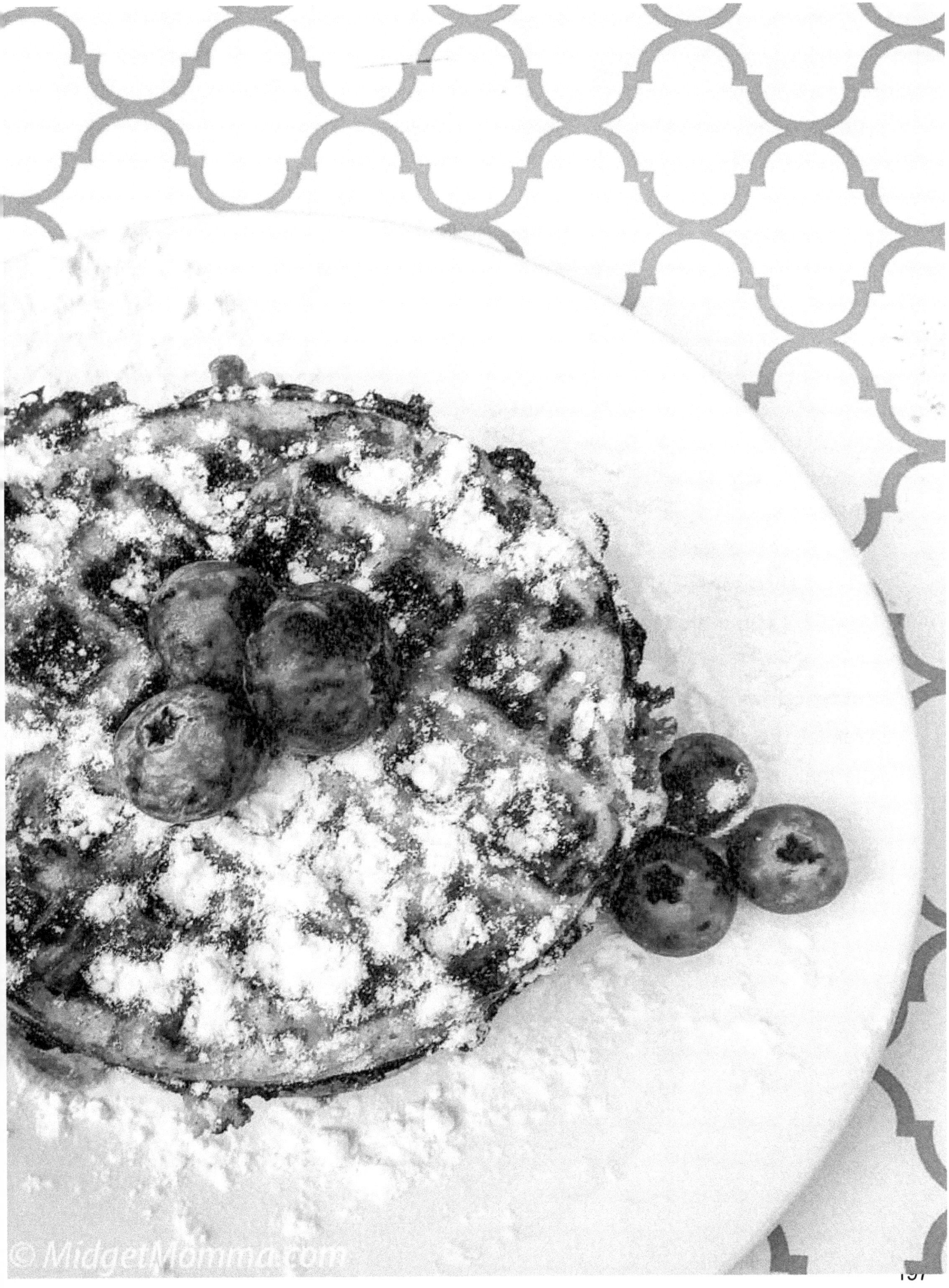
© MidgetMomma.com

33 Bread Sticks Chaffle

(Ready in about 12 minutes | Serving 7 | Difficulty: Easy)

Per serving: Kcal 80, Fat: 7g, Net Carbs: 1g, Protein: 5g

Ingredients

- 1 egg
- 2 tbsp of almond flour
- 1/2 cup grated mozzarella cheese
- 1/2tsp of garlic powder
- 1/2tsp of salt
- 1/2tsp of oregano

Topping

- 1/2tsp of garlic powder
- 2 tbsp softened butter
- 1/4 cup grated mozzarella cheese

Instructions

Preheat the maker and oil it. Mix all ingredients except topping ingredients. Pour in the maker and cook for around 5 minutes. Make four strips of waffle. Mix butter and garlic powder and coat strips with it. Sprinkle with mozzarella and cook for around 3 minutes.

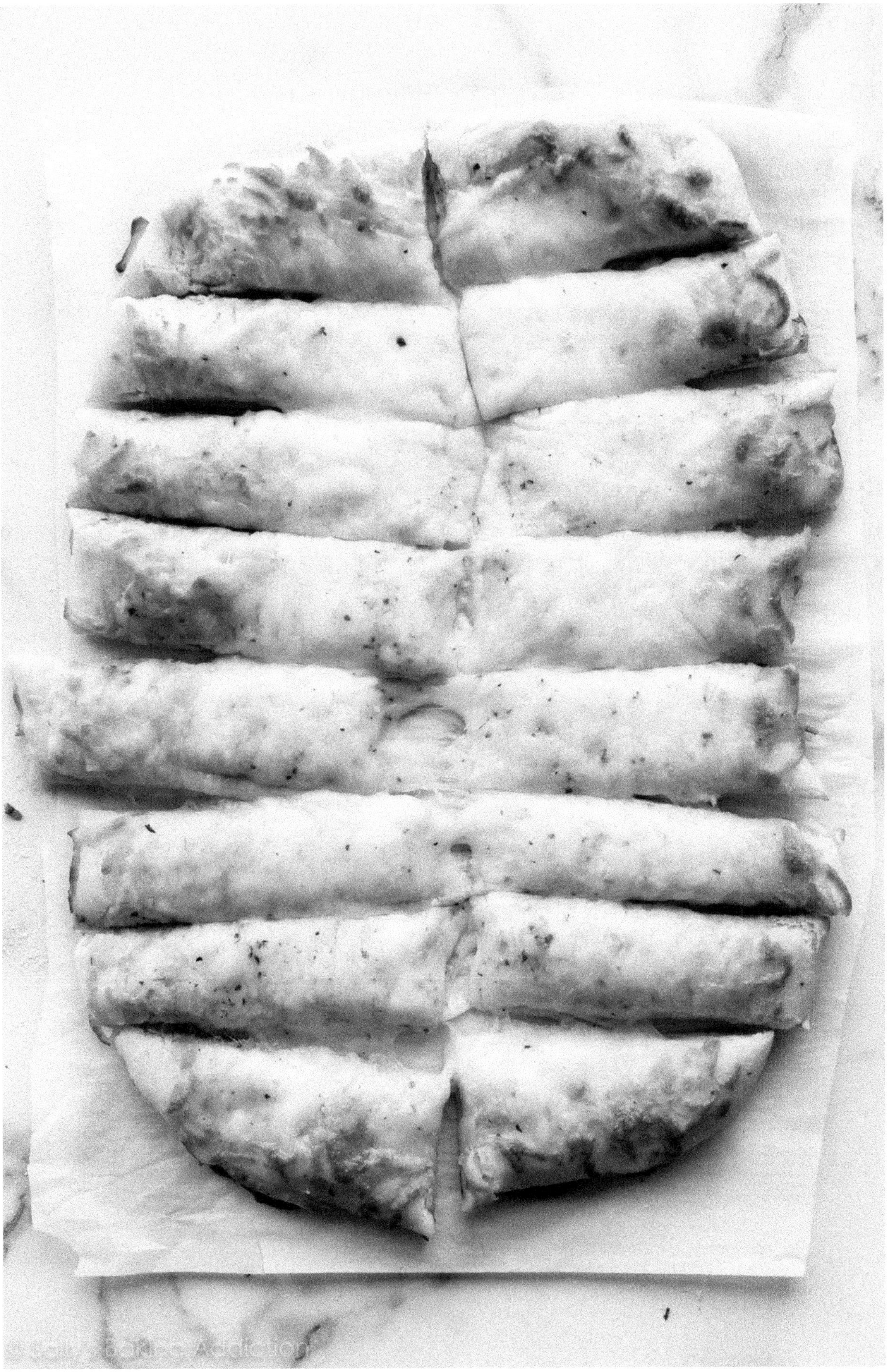

34 Original Chaffle

(Ready in about 5 minutes | Serving 1 | Difficulty: Easy)

Per serving: Kcal 246, Fat: 18g, Net Carbs: 2g, Protein: 17g

Ingredients

- 2 eggs
- 1/4 cup of almond flour
- 1/2 cup of mozzarella
- 1/2 tsp of baking powder

Instructions

Preheat iron and spray with cooking spray. Mix all the ingredients in a bowl and pour half amount of the mixture into the maker. Cook for around 5 minutes and repeat with the rest of the mixture.

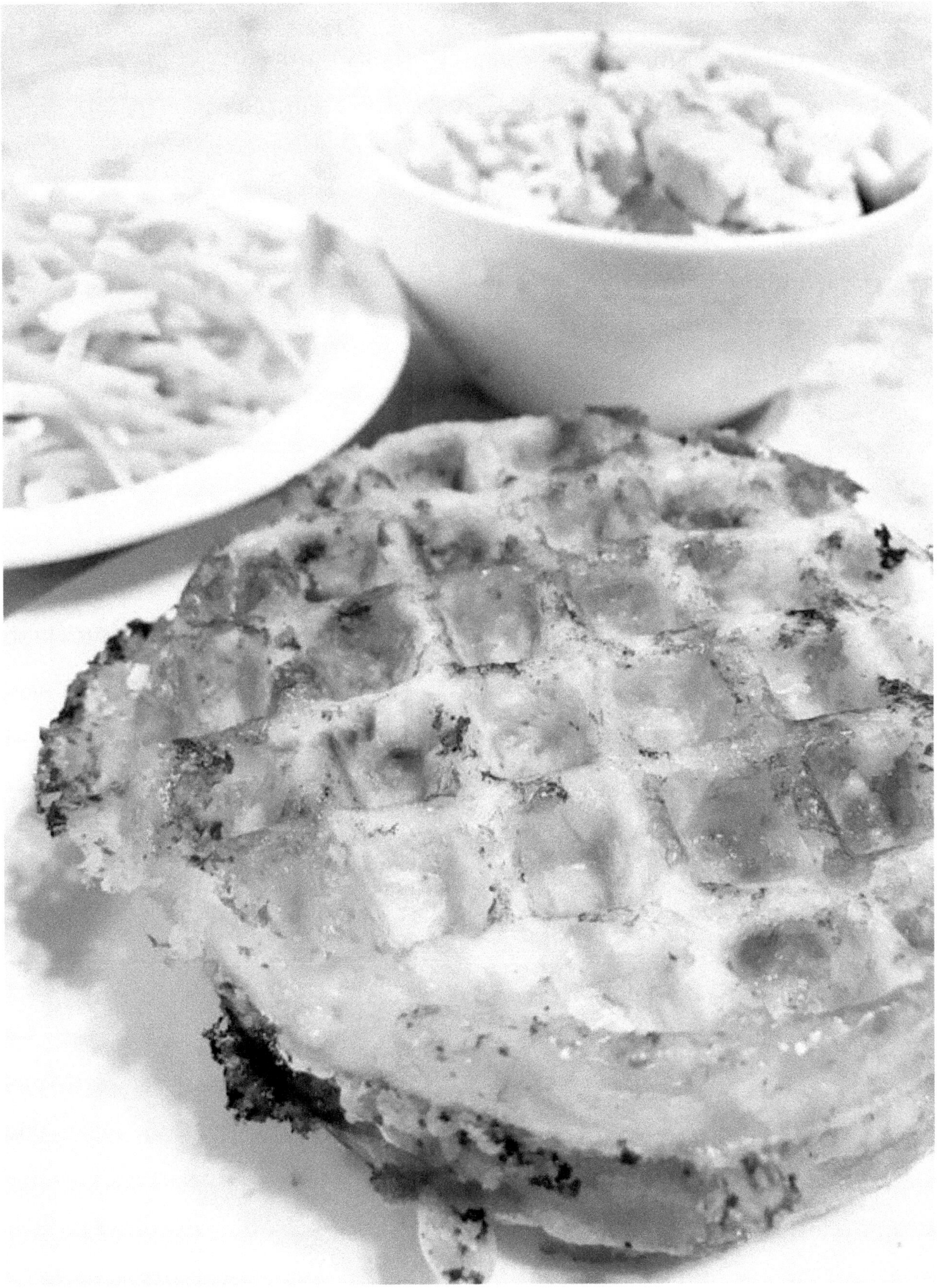

35 Mini Chaffles

(Ready in about 11 minutes | Serving 2 | Difficulty: Easy)

Per serving: Kcal 73, Fat: 6g, Net Carbs: 4g, Protein: 2g

Ingredients

- 2 tsp of Coconut Flour
- 1/4 tsp of Baking Powder
- 4 tsp of Swerve
- 1 Egg
- 1/2 tsp of Vanilla Extract
- 1 oz of Cream Cheese

Instructions

Preheat the iron. Add baking powder, coconut flour and swerve in a bowl and mix. Add cream cheese, egg and vanilla extract in bowl and mix. Pour mixture in the maker and cook for around 4 minutes.

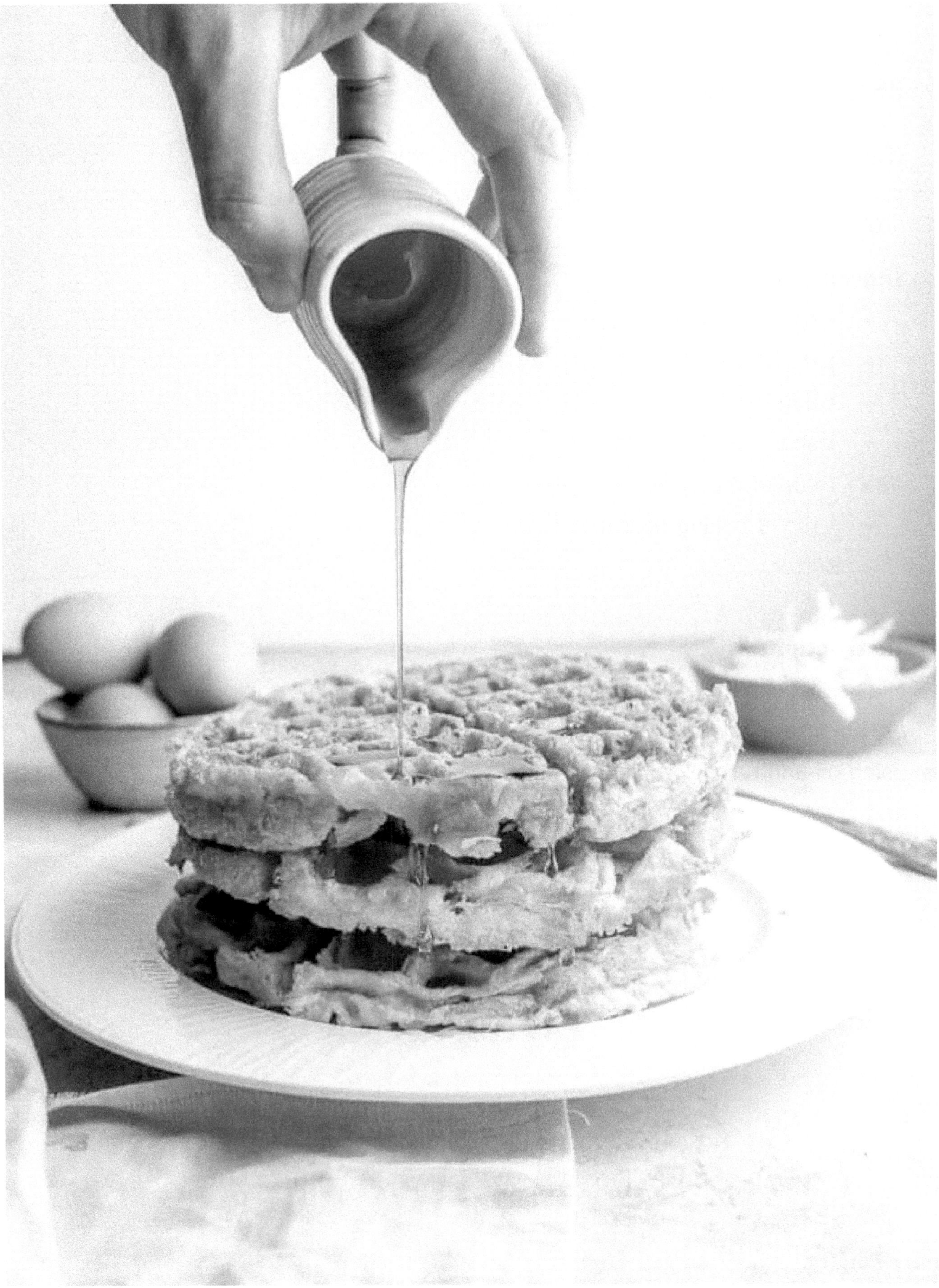

36 Grain-free chaffles

(Ready in about 20 minutes | Serving 2 | Difficulty: Easy)

Per serving: Kcal 277, Fat: 20g, Net Carbs: 4.6g, Protein: 4.8g

Ingredients

- 1 tbsp of almond flour
- 1 tsp of vanilla
- 1 egg
- 1 shake of cinnamon
- 1 cup of mozzarella cheese
- 1 tsp of baking powder
- Butter

Instructions

Mix vanilla extract and egg in a bowl. Mix almond flour, baking powder and cinnamon. Add mozzarella cheese at the end and coat with the mixture evenly. Spray waffle using oil and turn it on. Pour mixture and cook for around 5 minutes. Top with butter and enjoy.

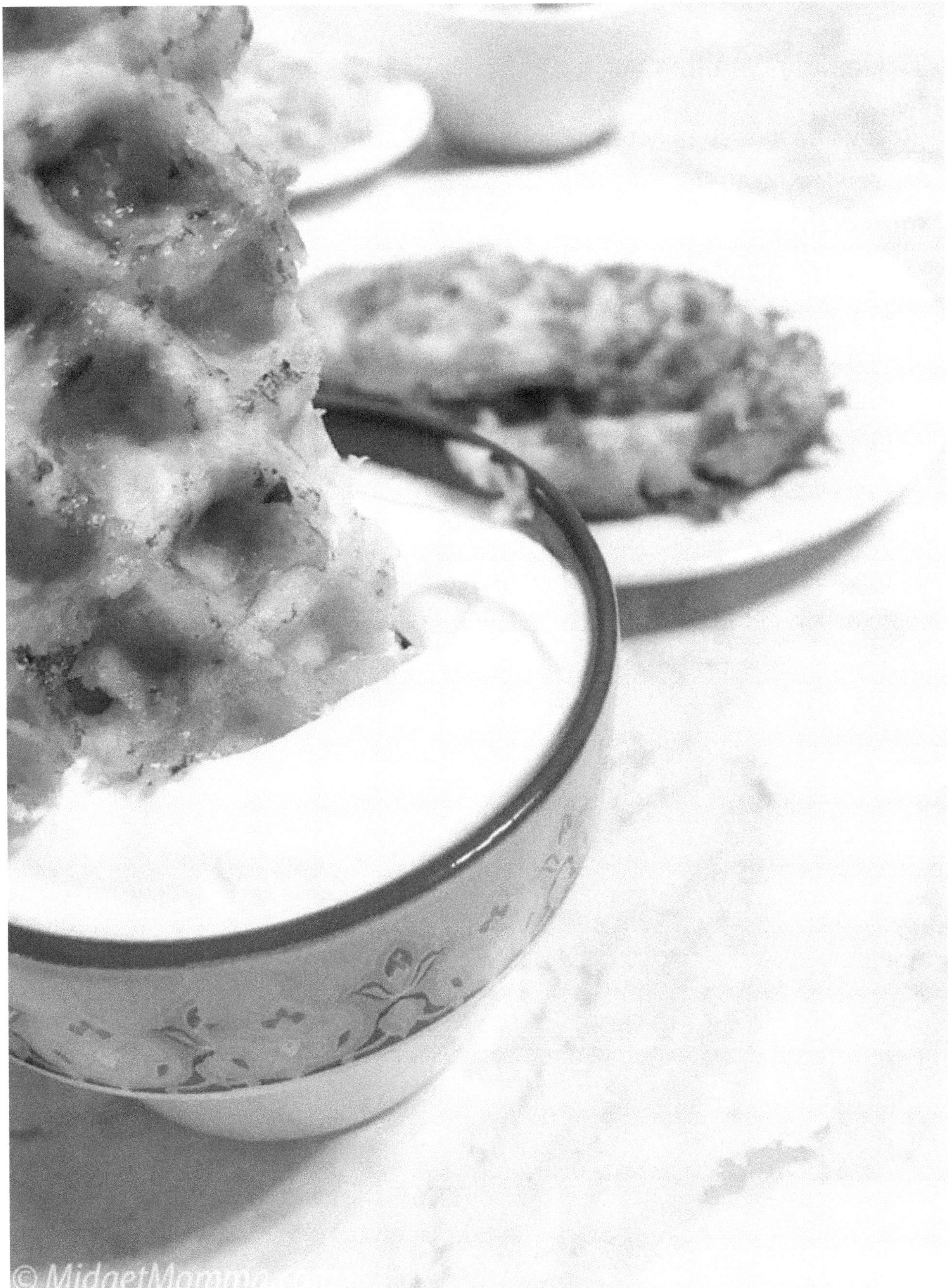
© MidgetMomma.com

37 Healthy Chaffles

(Ready in about 20 minutes | Serving 4 | Difficulty: Easy)

Per serving: Kcal 411, Fat: 35g, Net Carbs: 6g, Protein: 21g

Ingredients

- 1 1/2 cup of shredded cheese cheddar
- 4 oz. cream cheese
- 4 eggs
- 2 tsp of baking powder
- 1/2 cup of almond flour
- Syrup

Instructions

Oil the waffle maker and mix all ingredients in a bowl. Pour batter into the maker and cook for around 5 minutes. Top with syrup(sugar-free) and enjoy.

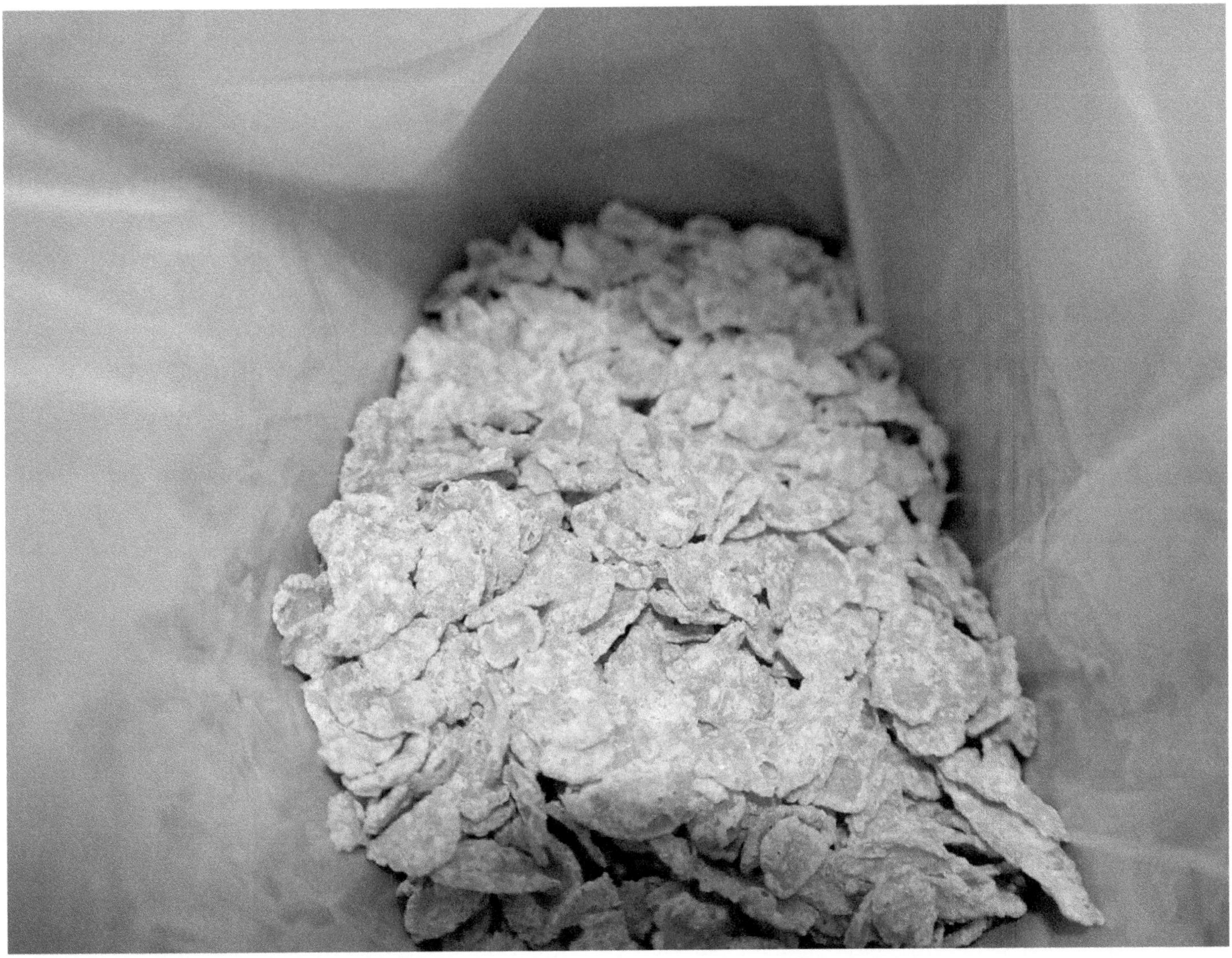

38 Sunny Chaffle

(Ready in about 10 minutes | Serving 1 | Difficulty: Easy)

Per serving: Kcal 320, Fat: 24.3g, Net Carbs: 3.1g, Protein: 21.7g

Ingredients

- 1 egg
- Strawberries
- 2 tbsp of almond flour
- 1/2 cup of mozzarella cheese
- 1/2tsp of baking powder

Instructions

Preheat the maker and mix all the ingredients in a bowl. Pour into the center of the maker and cook for around 5 minutes. Top with strawberries and enjoy.

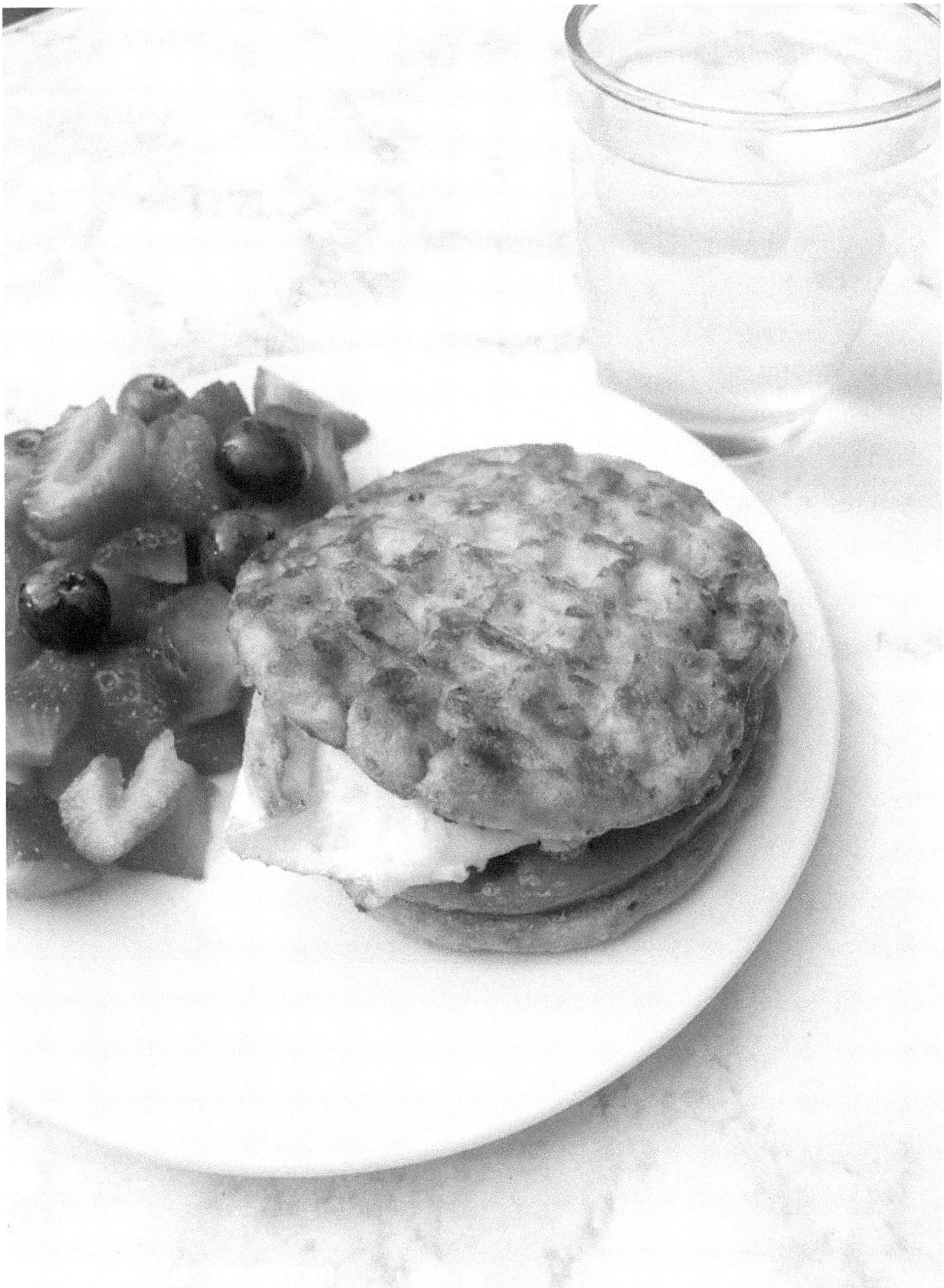

39 Traditional Chaffles

(Ready in about 13 minutes | Serving 1 | Difficulty: Easy)
Per serving: Kcal 291, Fat: 23g, Net Carbs: 1g, Protein: 20g

Ingredients

- 1/2 cup of shredded cheese cheddar
- 1 egg

Instructions

Preheat the maker and oil it gently. Break the egg in a bowl and add the half cup of cheddar cheese. Mix and pour half amount of mixture in maker. Cook for around 4 minutes. Repeat with the rest of the mixture.

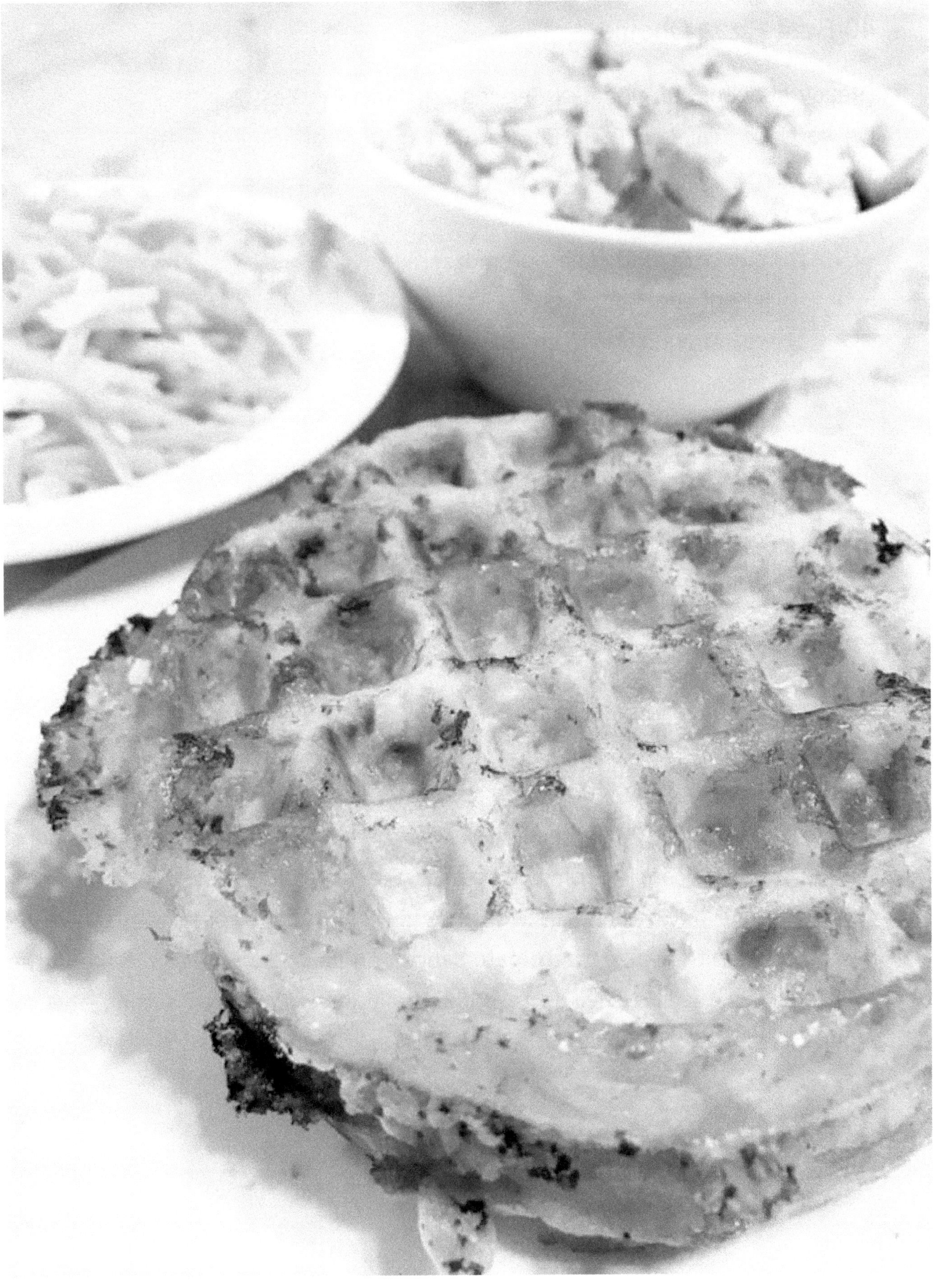

40 Best Pizza Chaffle

(Ready in about 20 minutes | Serving 2 | Difficulty: Easy)

Per serving: Kcal 241, Fat: 18g, Net Carbs: 4g, Protein: 17g

Ingredients

- 1 tsp of coconut flour
- 1/2 cup of shredded cheese mozzarella
- 1 white of egg
- `1 tsp softened cream cheese
- 1/8 tsp of Italian seasoning
- 1/4 tsp of baking powder
- 1/8 tsp of garlic powder
- 3 tsp of marinara sauce
- Salt
- 1/2 cup of mozzarella cheese
- 1 tbsp shredded cheese parmesan
- 6 pepperonis diced in half
- 1/4 tsp of basil seasoning

Instructions

Preheat the oven to 400 degrees F. Preheat the maker as well. Add all the ingredients except pepperoni and parmesan cheese in a bowl and mix. Pour half amount of mixture in the maker and cook for around 4 minutes. Repeat with the rest of the mixture. Top with pepperoni, tomato sauce and parmesan cheese. Bake in the oven by placing on the top shelf for around 6 minutes. Turn broil setting and cook for around 2 minutes. Sprinkle with basil.

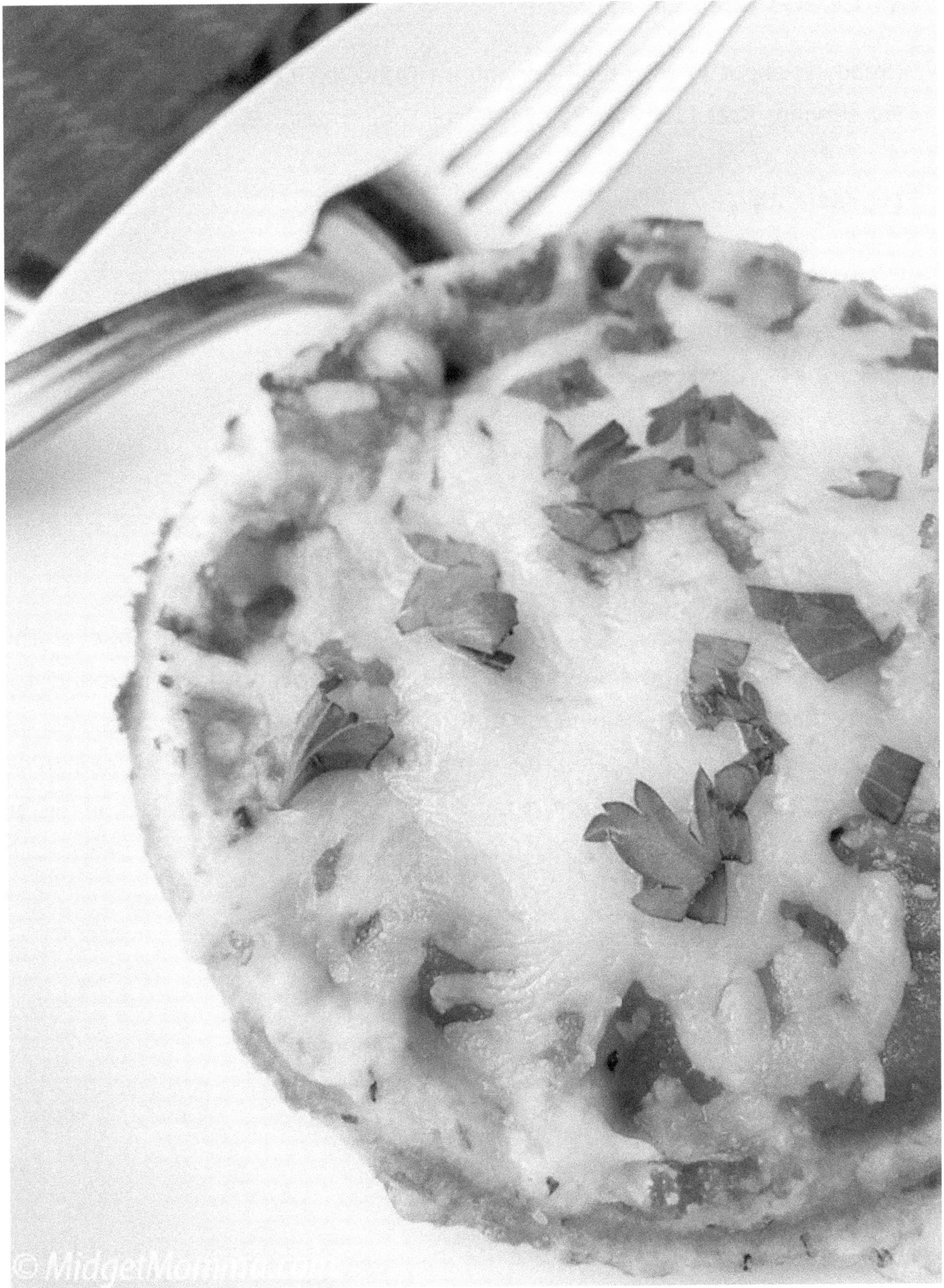
© MidgetMomma.com

41 Open-Faced Chaffle

(Ready in about 17 minutes | Serving 2 | Difficulty: Easy)
Per serving: Kcal 118, Fat: 8g, Net Carbs: 2g, Protein: 9g

Ingredients

- 1 egg only white
- 1/4 cup shredded cheddar cheese
- 1/4 cup shredded cheese mozzarella
- 3/4 tsp of water
- 1/4 tsp of baking powder
- 1 tsp of coconut flour
- Salt

Instructions

Preheat the oven to 425 degrees F. Preheat the maker as well. Mix everything in a bowl and pour half the amount of mixture into a maker. Cook for around 4 minutes and repeat with the remaining mixture. Line parchment paper on a cookie sheet and place chaffles on it. Add a quarter cup of roasted keto beef gravy. Add cheese slice on top and bake in the oven for around 5 minutes in the top rack. Broil for around 1 minute.

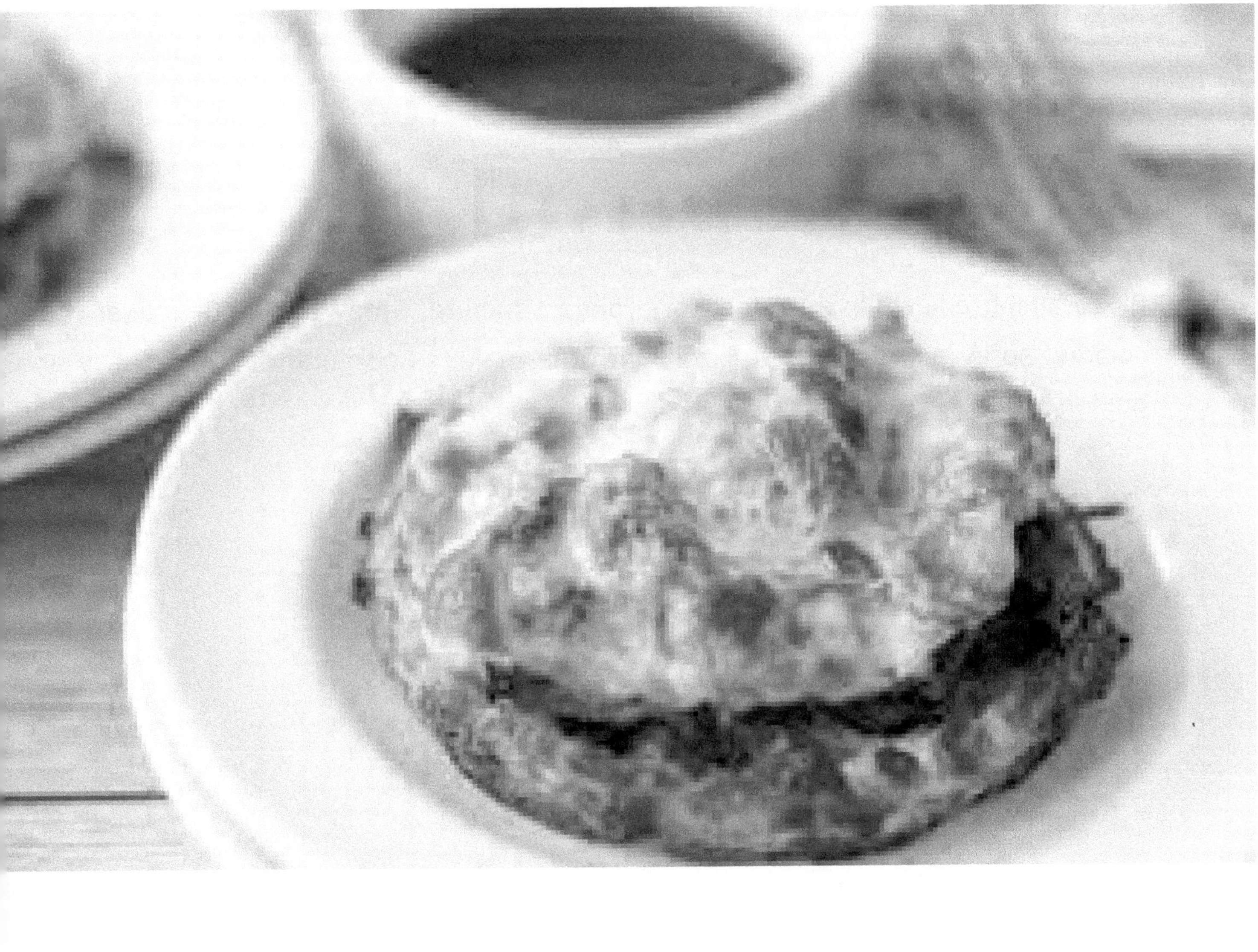

42 Cream Chaffles

(Ready in about 15 minutes | Serving 2 | Difficulty: Easy)
Per serving: Kcal 293, Fat: 27g, Net Carbs: 5g, Protein: 10g

Ingredients

- 4 eggs
- 1 tsp of vanilla extract
- 2 tbsp of melted butter
- 4 oz of cream cheese
- 1 tsp of baking powder

Instructions

Blend all ingredients in a blender for around 1 minute. Spray the waffle maker using cooking spray and pour the mixture into the maker. Cook until it turns crispy and golden.

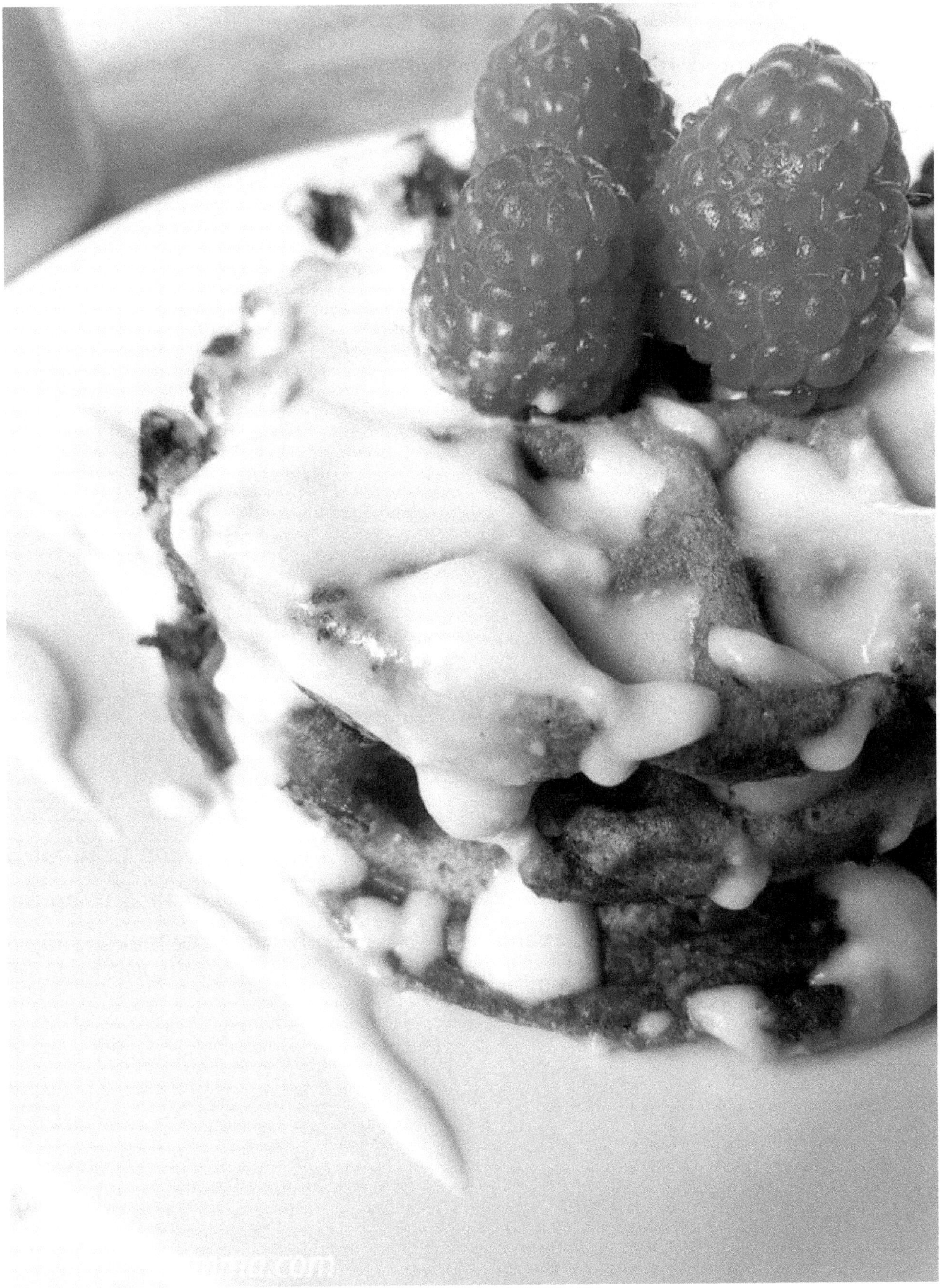

43 Fluffy Chaffles

(Ready in about 45 minutes | Serving 8 | Difficulty: Moderate)
Per serving: Kcal 140, Fat: 11g, Net Carbs: 4g, Protein: 4g

Ingredients

- 64 g of almond flour
- 1 1/2 tsp of baking powder
- 1 tbsp of ground psyllium husk
- 28 g of coconut flour
- 1 tsp of xanthan gum
- 57 g of butter
- 240 ml of water
- 3 tbsp of erythritol
- 3 eggs beaten
- 1/4 tsp of kosher salt
- 1 tsp of vanilla extract

Instructions

Mix flours, xantham gum and husk in a bowl. Warm water, sweetener, salt and butter in a pot and once it starts simmering, add flours and incorporate. Cook for around 3 minutes. Transfer dough to bowl and add egg one by one, mixing using an electric mixer. Add baking powder and vanilla extract and mix. Heat the maker and oil it. Pour batter and cook for around 12 minutes.

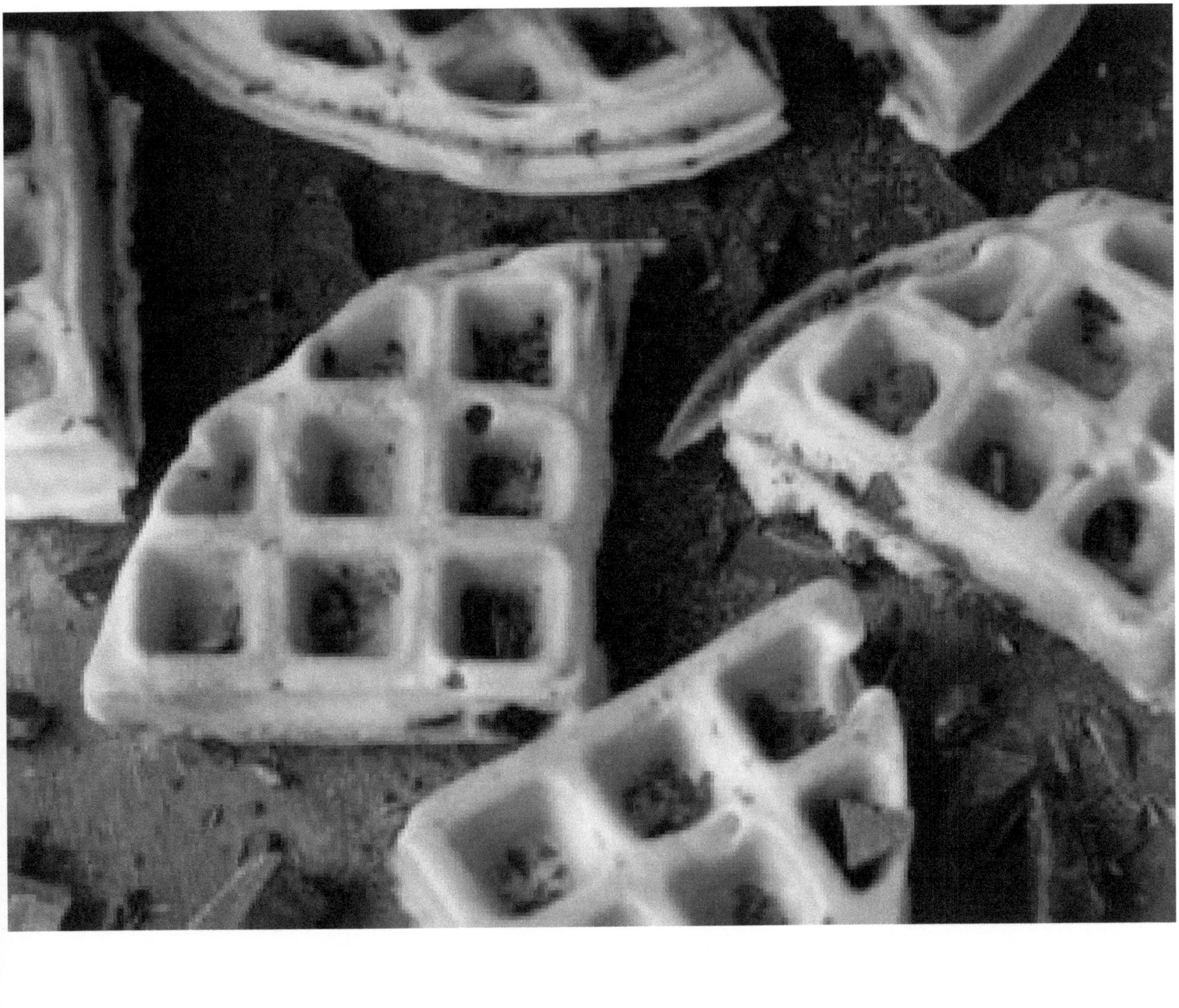

44 Almond Flour Chaffles

(Ready in about 20 minutes | Serving 2 | Difficulty: Easy)

Per serving: Kcal 70, Fat: 3.8g, Net Carbs: 4.9g, Protein: 4g

Ingredients

- 4 separated eggs
- 1/4 cup of granulated Swerve
- 2 cup of almond flour
- 2 tsp of baking powder
- 1/2 cup of butter
- 1 tsp of kosher salt
- 1/2 cup of almond butter
- Cooking spray
- 2 tsp. of vanilla extract
- Maple syrup

Instructions

Preheat waffle maker to high. Mix stevia, almond flour, salt and baking powder in a bowl. Melt almond butter and butter in the microwave for around 15 seconds. Stir dry ingredients with butter mixture and then add vanilla and yolks. Beat whites in a separate bowl and fold in batter. Spray maker using cooking spray and pour the batter. Cook for around 5 minutes. Top with maple syrup and butter.

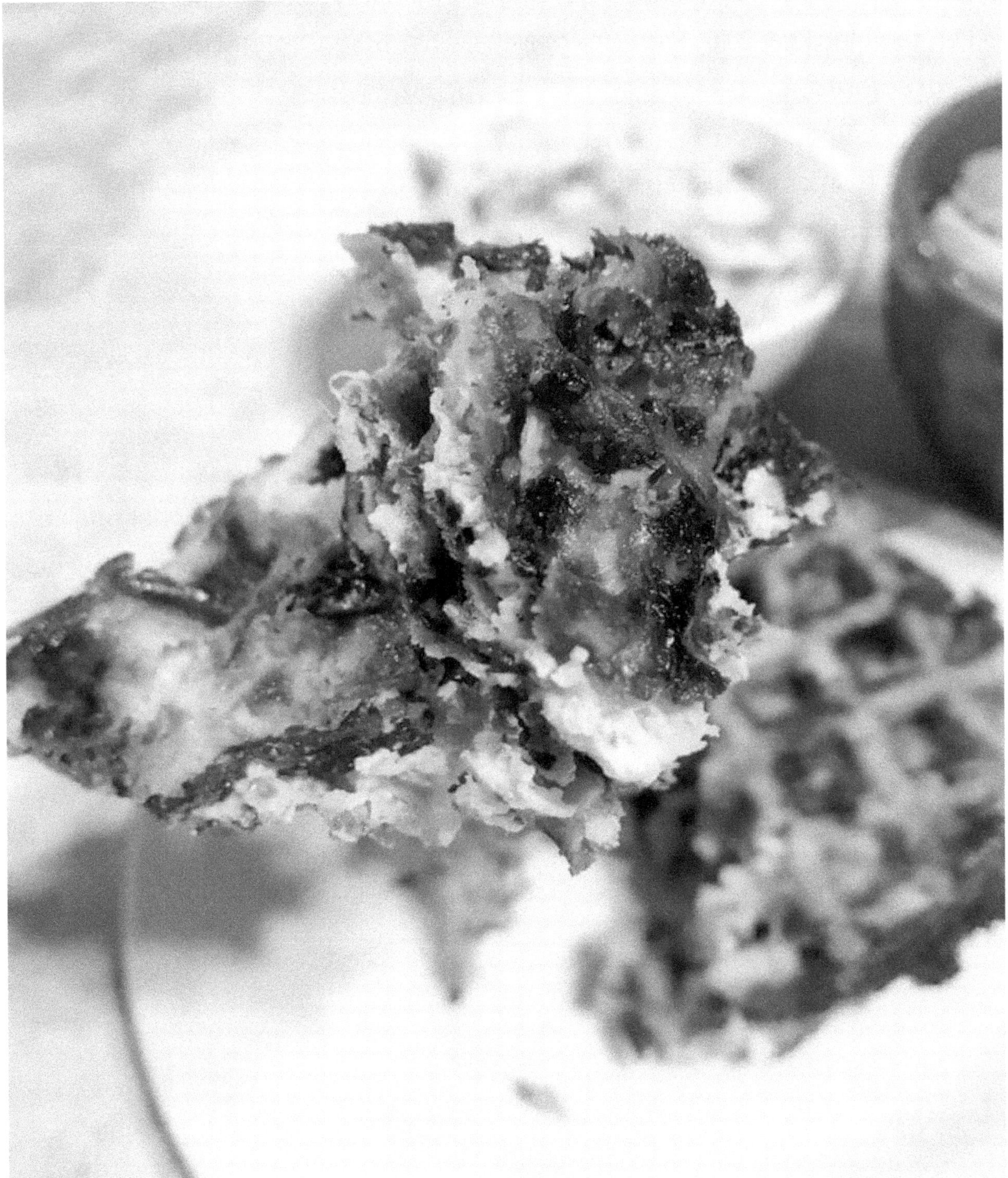

45 Butter Chaffles

(Ready in about 30 minutes | Serving 5 | Difficulty: Easy)

Per serving: Kcal 216, Fat: 19.9g, Net Carbs: 5.5g, Protein: 6.4g

Ingredients

- 5 eggs
- 4 tbsp of granulated sweetener
- 4 tbsp of coconut flour
- 1 tsp of baking powder
- 3 tbsp of milk full fat
- 2 tsp of vanilla
- 125 g of butter melted

Instructions

Beat egg whites in a bowl. Mix yolks with sweetener, baking powder and coconut flour in a separate bowl. Add butter and mix. Add vanilla and milk and mix. Fold whites in yolk mixture and pour in maker. Cook for around 5 minutes.

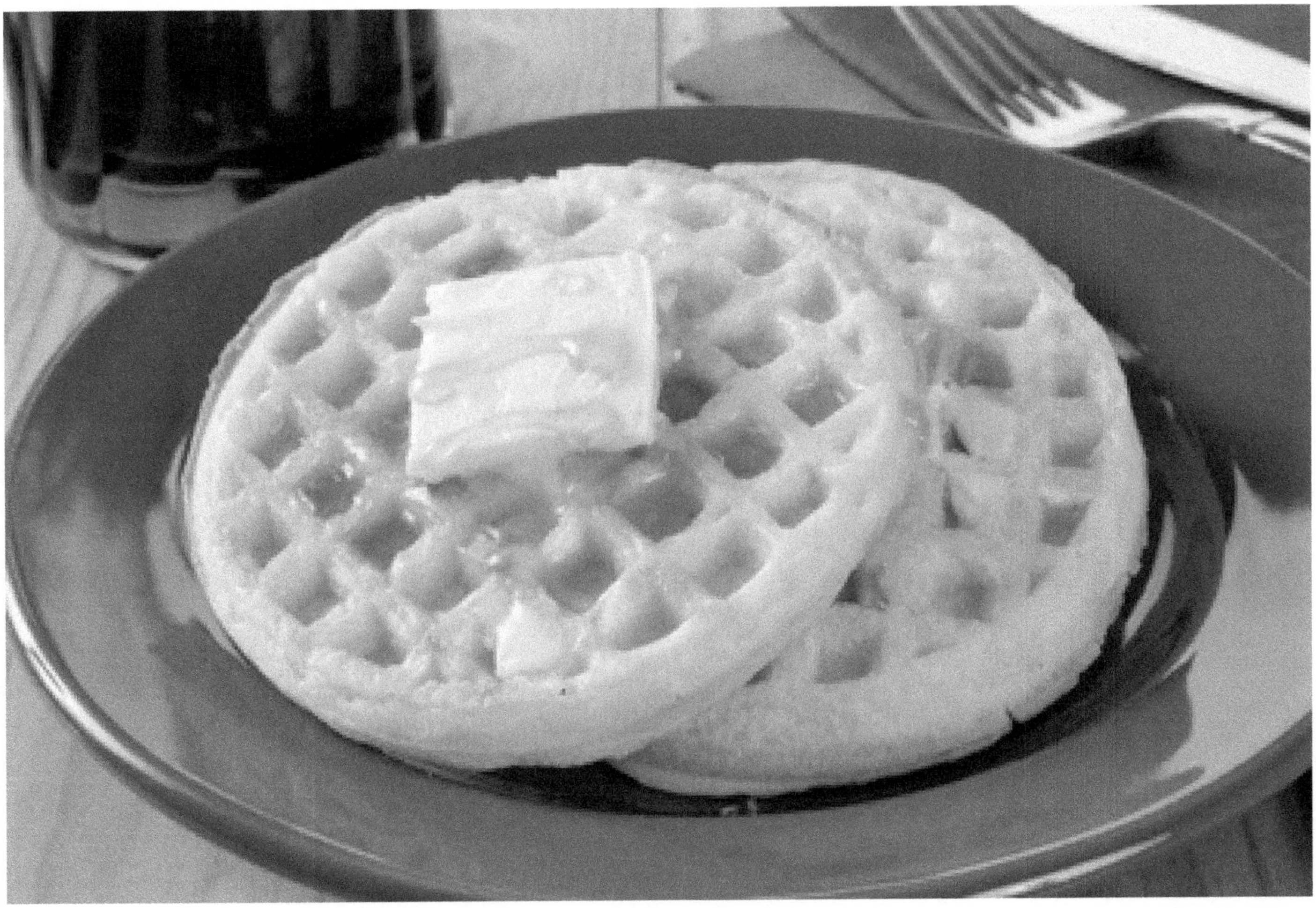

46 Paleo Chaffles

(Ready in about 10minutes | Serving 2 | Difficulty: Easy)

Per serving: Kcal 401, Fat: 37, Net Carbs: 9g, Protein: 13g

Ingredients

- 1 egg
- 2 tbsp of sweetener
- 1/2 cup of Almond Flour
- 1/2 tsp of baking powder Gluten-free
- 2 tbsp of Almond butter
- 1/4 tsp of Sea salt
- 2 tbsp of Butter
- 1/2 tsp of Vanilla extract
- 1/4 cup of almond milk Unsweetened

Instructions

Preheat waffle maker to high temperature. Oil it gently and beat whites in a bowl. Combine baking powder, erythritol, salt and almond flour in another bowl. Melt almond butter and butter in the microwave and add to the flour mixture. Add yolk, vanilla and almond milk and stir. Fold whites in batter and mix. Pour in the maker and cook for around 5 minutes.

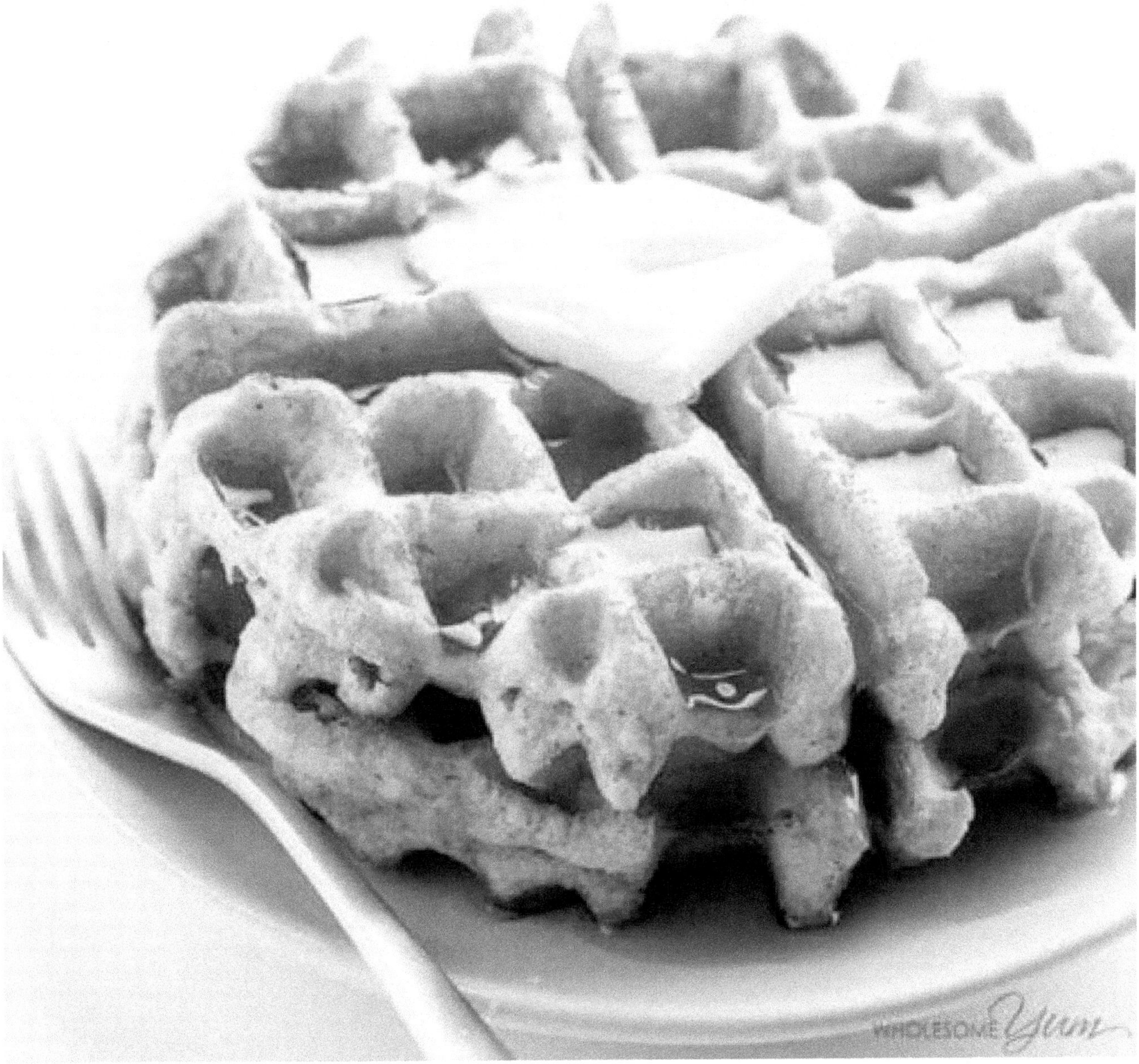
WHOLESOME Yum

47 Crispy Chaffles

(Ready in about 10 minutes | Serving 4 | Difficulty: Easy)

Per serving: Kcal 64, Fat: 2g, Net Carbs: 4g, Protein: 5g

Ingredients

- 4 tbsp sifted coconut flour
- 1/4 tsp of baking powder
- 1 tsp of coconut oil
- 1 tbsp sweetener granulated
- 2/3 cup of egg whites
- 1/2 tsp of vanilla extract
- 1/4 cup of milk
- 1 tbsp of unsweetened apple sauce

Instructions

Mix sweetener, baking powder and coconut flour in a bowl. Add whites, vanilla, apple sauce and milk in a separate bowl and mix. Pour to the other bowl and form a thick batter. Add oil and spray waffle maker using cooking spray. Once the maker is hot, pour the batter and cook for around 4 minutes.

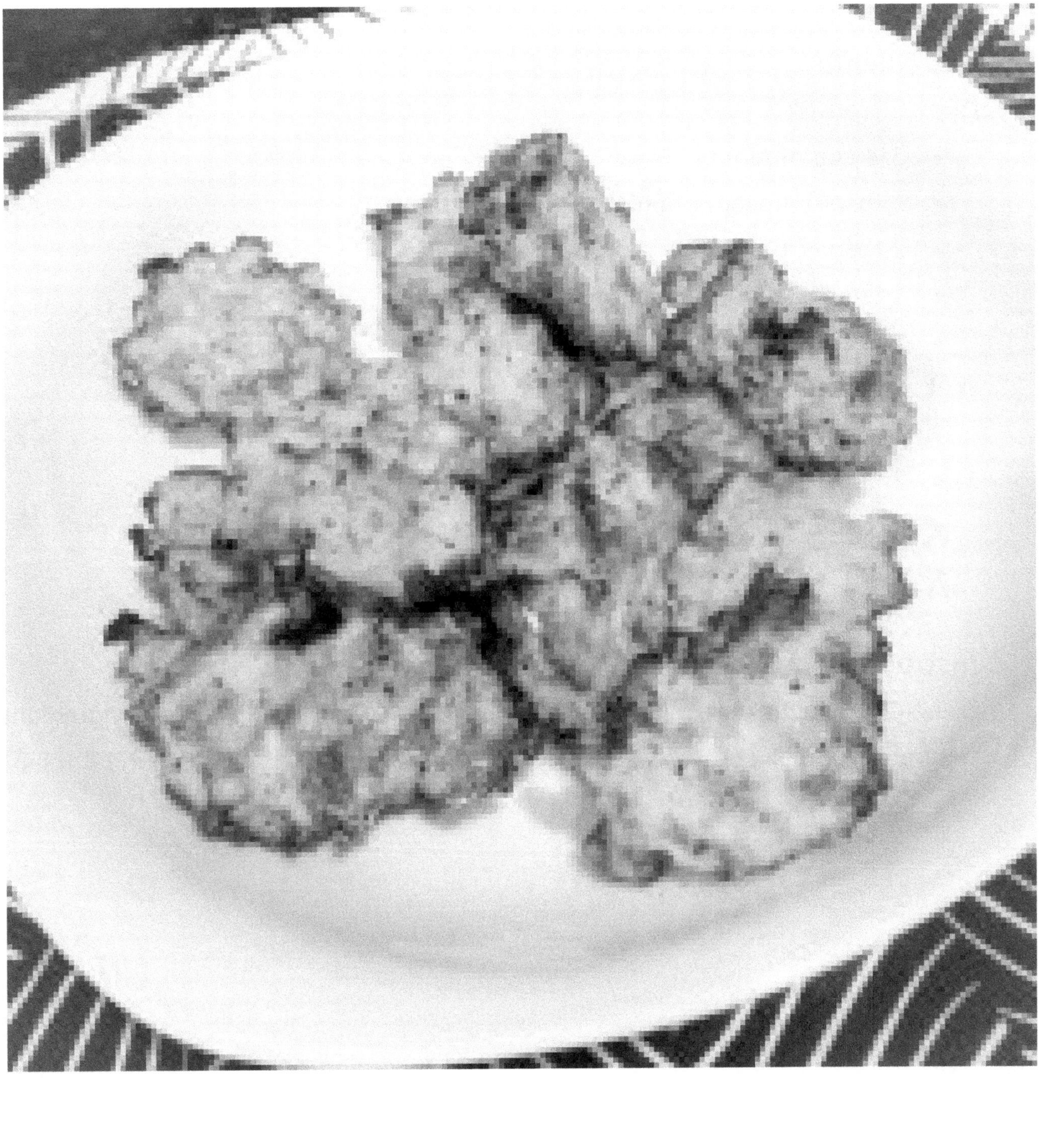

48 Salted Chaffles

(Ready in about 15 minutes | Serving 2 | Difficulty: Easy)

Per serving: Kcal 425, Fat: 36.7g, Net Carbs: 10.7g, Protein: 14.8g

Ingredients

Dry

- 3/4 cup of Almond Flour
- 1 tbsp of Coconut flour
- 2 tbsp of Erythritol
- 1 tsp of Baking Powder
- 1/8 tsp of Himalayan Salt

Wet

- 2 tbsp of Melted Butter
- 2 Eggs
- 2 tbsp of Cream Cheese at room temperature
- 1 tsp of Vanilla Extract

Instructions

Preheat waffle maker to high. Mix wet ingredients in a bowl. Mix dry ingredients in a separate bowl. Mix both bowls and pour in the maker. Cook for around 4 minutes.

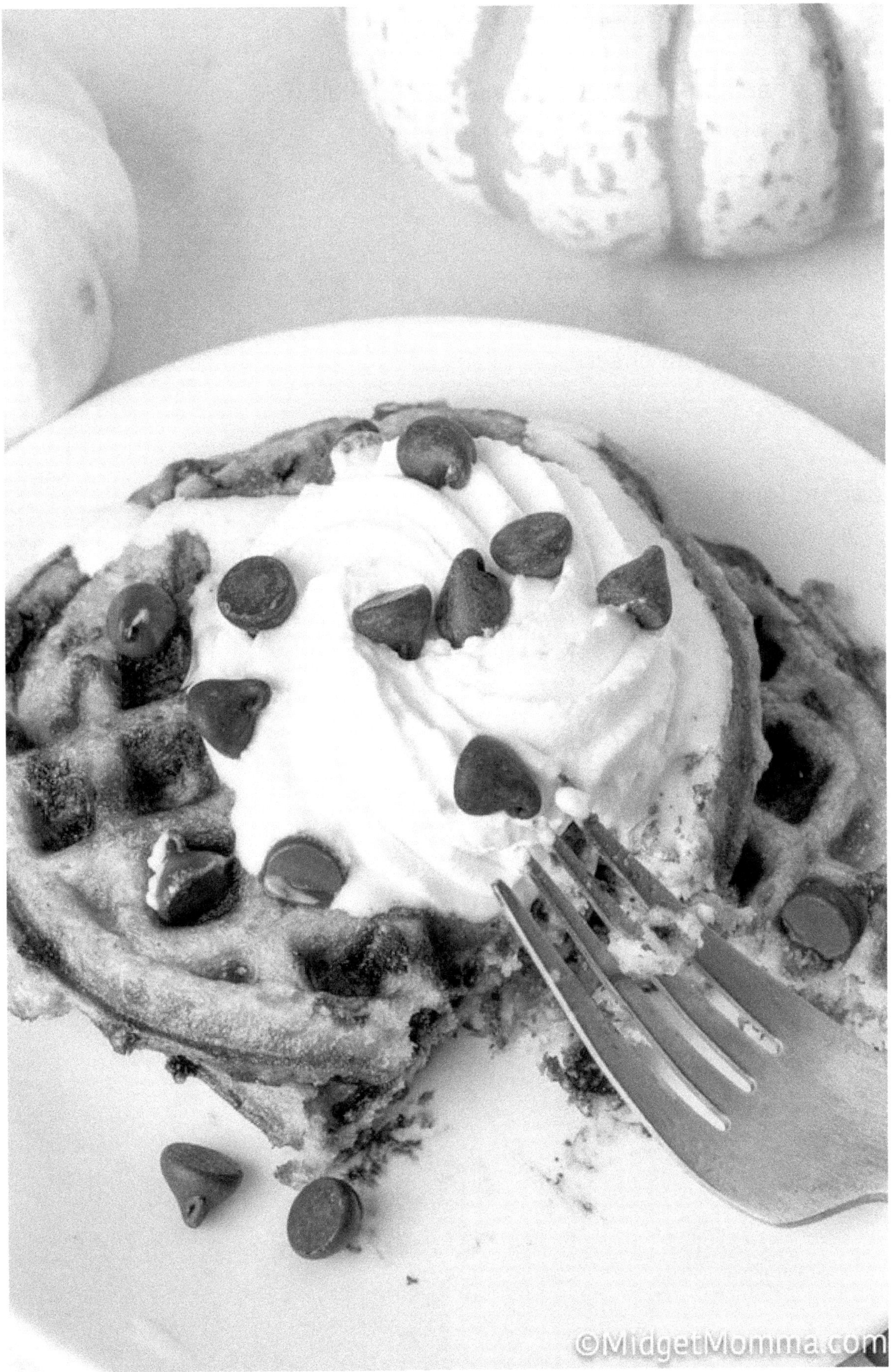
©MidgetMomma.com

49 Low Carb Chaffles

(Ready in about 8 minutes | Serving 1 | Difficulty: Easy)

Per serving: Kcal 522, Fat: 48g, Net Carbs: 7g, Protein: 19g

Ingredients

- 2 eggs
- 1/2 tsp of baking powder
- 4 tbsp of almond flour
- 2 oz of cream cheese
- 1 tbsp of coconut oil

Instructions

Blend everything in the blender and pour in the maker, which is oiled. Cook for around 3 minutes.

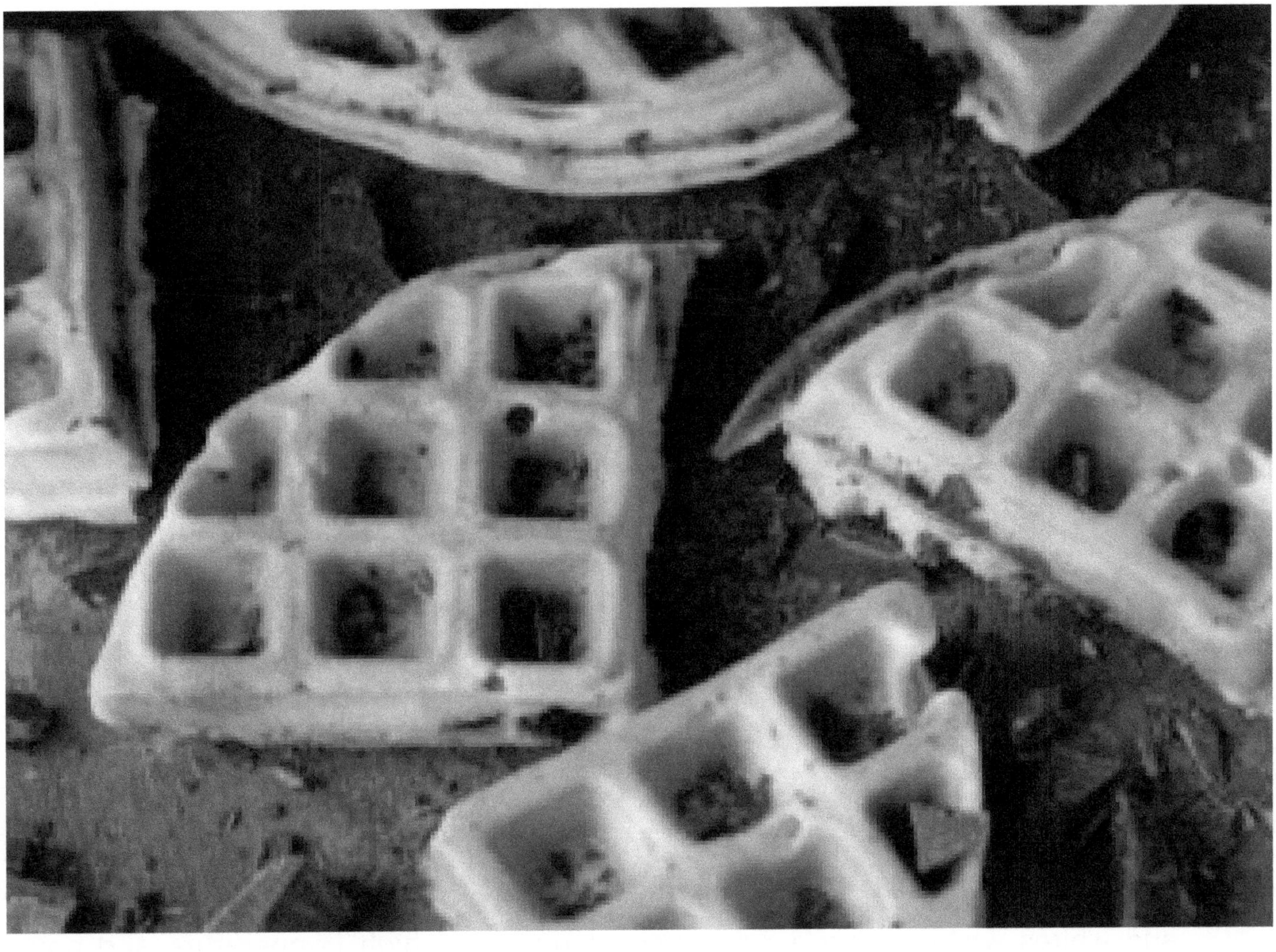

50 Sweet Chaffles

(Ready in about 9 minutes | Serving 2 | Difficulty: Easy)

Per serving: Kcal 331, Fat: 29g, Net Carbs: 7g, Protein: 11g

Ingredients

Dry

- 1/2 cup of almond flour
- 1/2 tsp of sweetener
- 1/4tsp of baking soda
- 1/4tsp of salt
- 1/4 tsp of baking powder
- 1/8 tsp of nutmeg
- 1/4tsp of ground cinnamon
- 1/8 tsp of cloves

Wet

- 2 eggs
- 2 tbsp of melted butter
- 1 tsp of vanilla extract

Instructions

Add dry ingredients to a bowl and mix. Separate yolks and whites in two bowls and mix butter and vanilla in yolks. Beat whites and add yolks to dry ingredients. Then add whites while mixing gently. Preheat maker to high temperature and pour the mixture. Cook for around 5 minutes.

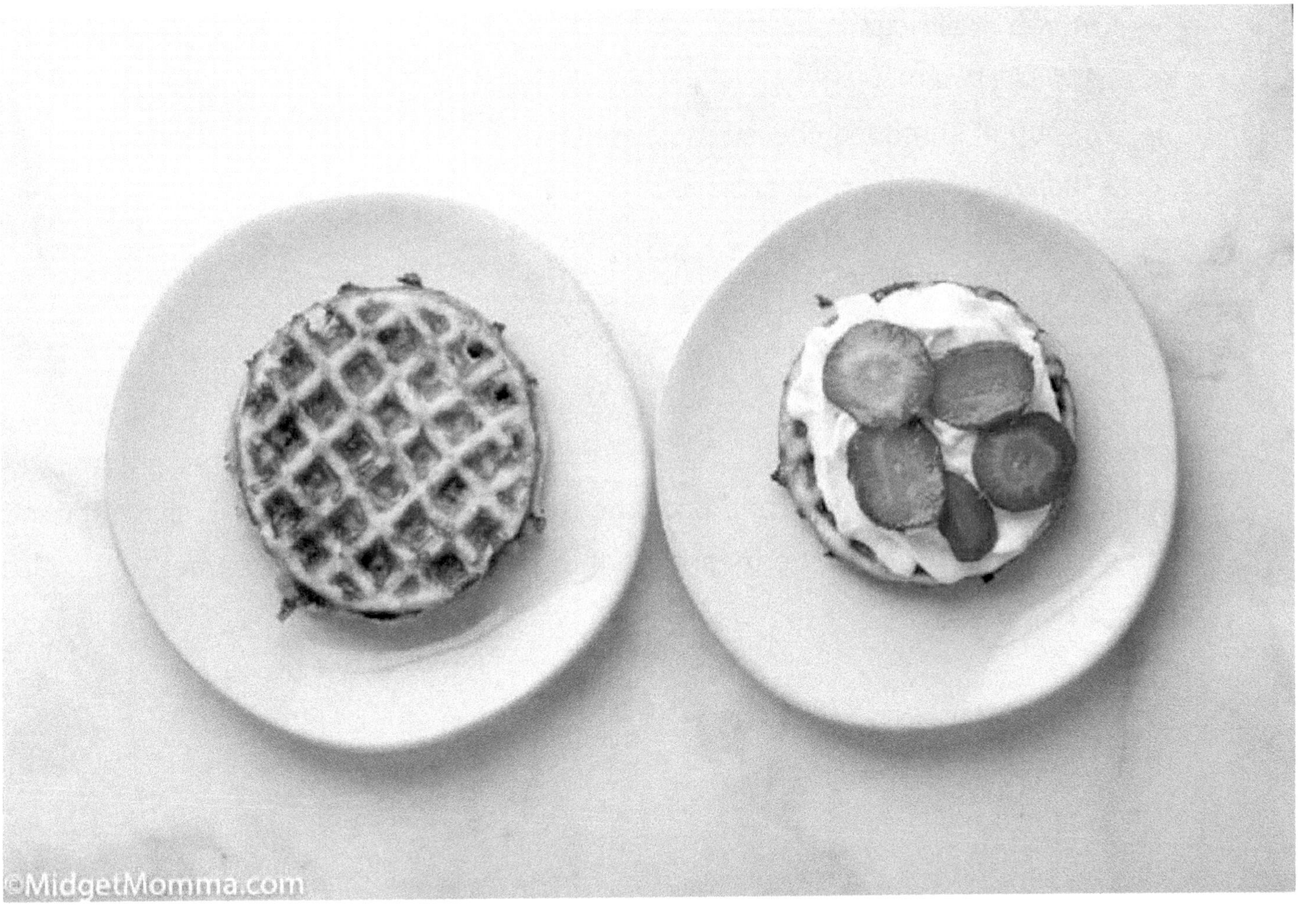
©MidgetMomma.com

51 Churro Chaffle

(Ready in about 15 minutes | Serving 1 | Difficulty: Easy)

Per serving: Kcal 193, Fat: 14g, Net Carbs: 2g, Protein: 8g

Ingredients

- 1 egg
- 1/4 cup of almond flour
- 1 tsp of cinnamon
- 1/2 cup of shredded cheese mozzarella
- 2 tbsp of Swerve granular
- 2 tbsp of melted butter
- ⅛ tsp of baking powder
- 3 tbsp of Swerve granular

Instructions

Combine everything in a bowl and pour the mixture into the maker by dividing it into three parts. Melt butter in the meantime in a pan over moderate flame. Add churro toppings and enjoy.

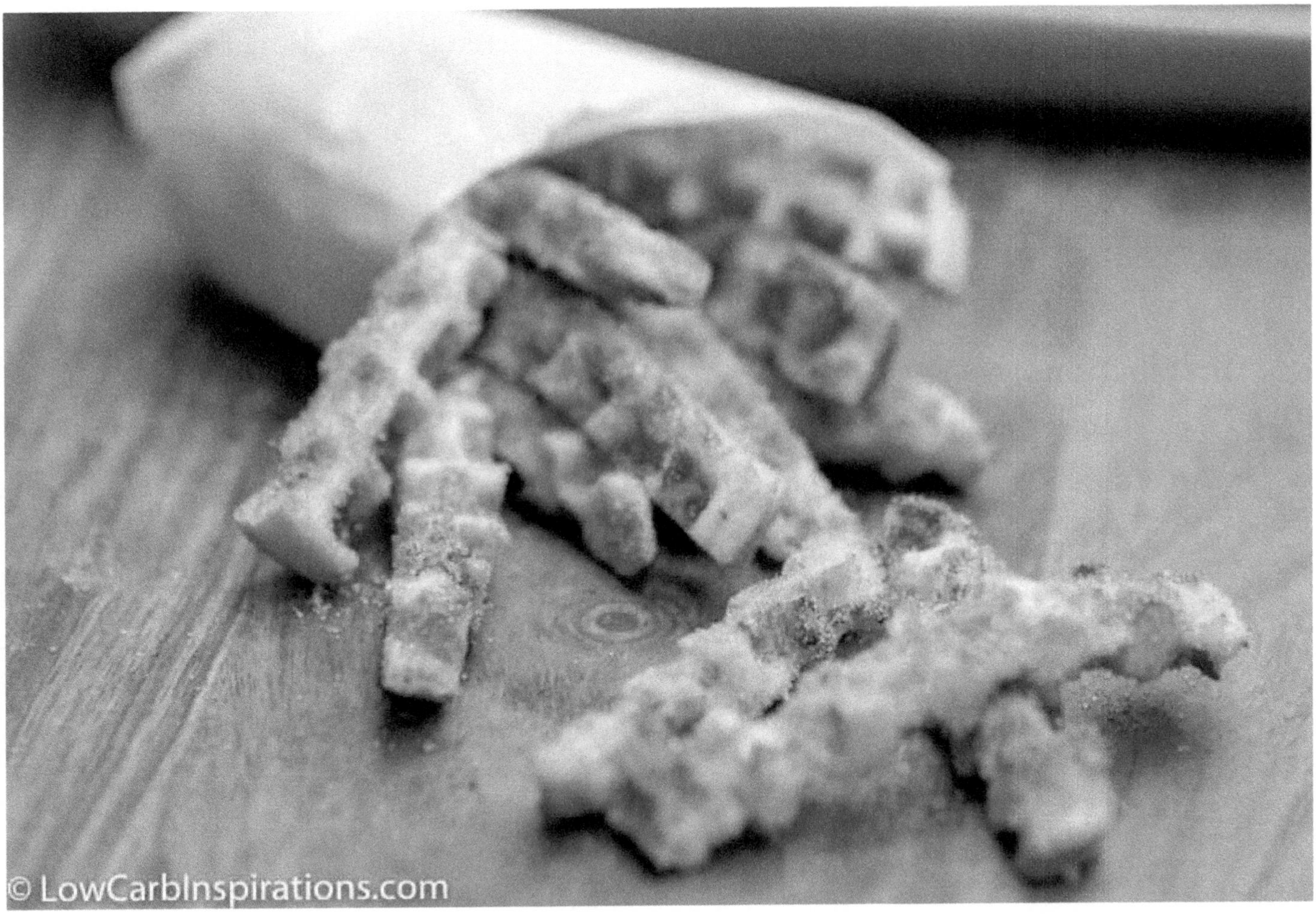
© LowCarbInspirations.com

52 Avocado Egg Bake

(Ready in about 20 minutes | Serving 1 | Difficulty: Easy)

Per serving: Kcal 605, Fat: 50.9g, Net Carbs: 18.6g, Protein: 25.3g

Ingredients

- 2 eggs
- 1 avocado, pitted and halved
- ¼ cup of shredded Cheddar cheese
- 1 tbsp. chopped fresh parsley, or according to taste
- Freshly ground black pepper and salt according to taste

Instructions

- Preheat oven to 425 degrees Fahrenheit.
- To make way for one egg, scoop out some of the avocados from where the pit. Put each avocado half on the baking sheet, then crack one egg on top.
- Cook for fifteen to twenty minutes in a preheated oven before the egg is ready. Season with pepper and salt and finish with Cheddar cheese. Serve with new parsley as a garnish.

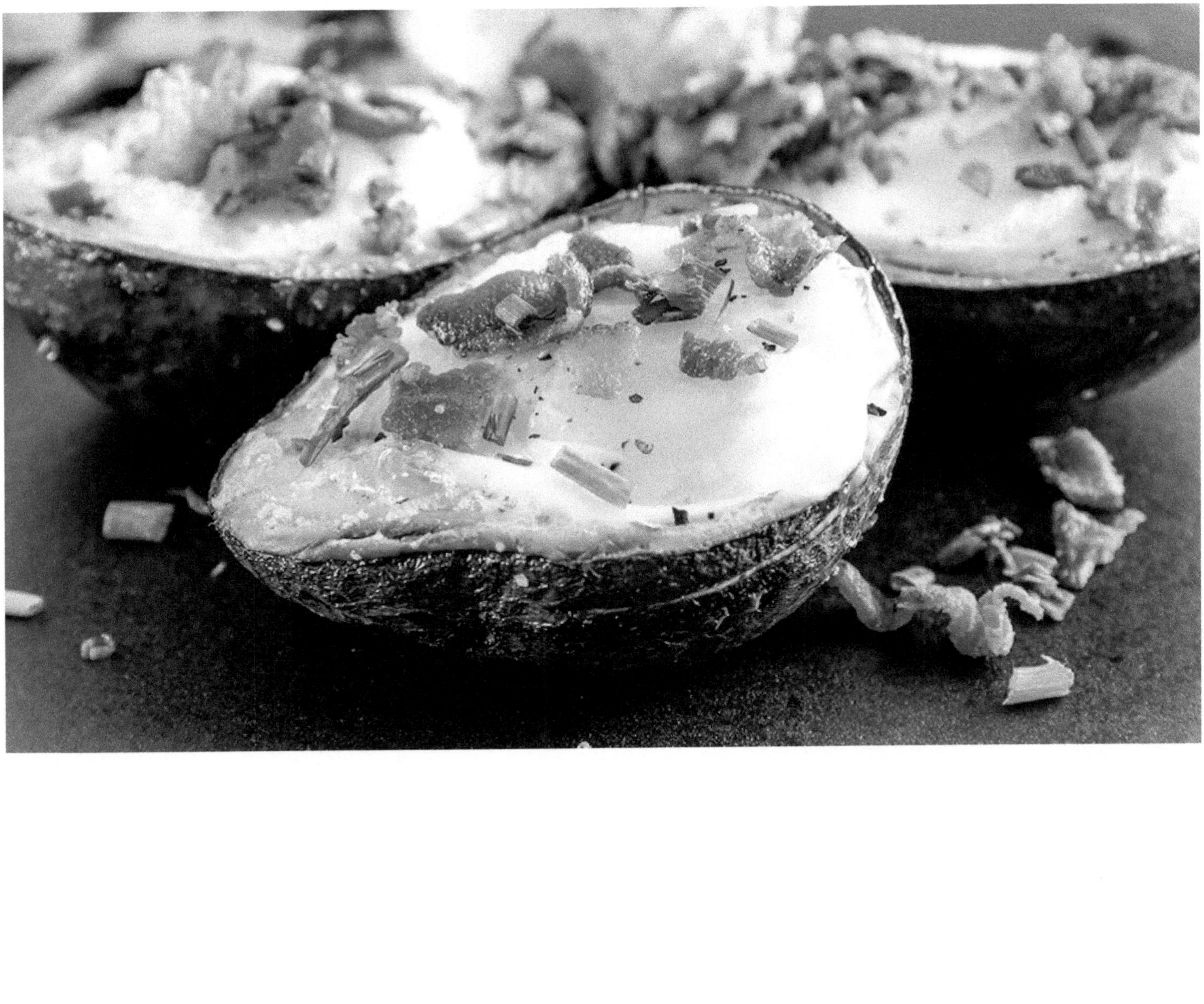

53 Oven-Baked Bacon

(Ready in about 35 minutes | Serving 6 | Difficulty: Easy)

Per serving: Kcal 134, Fat: 10.4g, Net Carbs: 0.4g, Protein: 9.2g

Ingredients

1 (16 oz.) package bacon

Instructions

- Preheat oven to 350°F. Using parchment paper, line a baking dish.
- Put the bacon slices on a prepared baking sheet, one on top of the other.
- Bake for fifteen to twenty minutes in a preheated oven. Take off the dish from the oven. Return the bacon slices to the oven after tossing them with kitchen tongs. Bake for another fifteen to twenty minutes, or till crispy. Thinner slices may require less time to cook, about twenty minutes overall. Drain on a paper towel-lined pan.

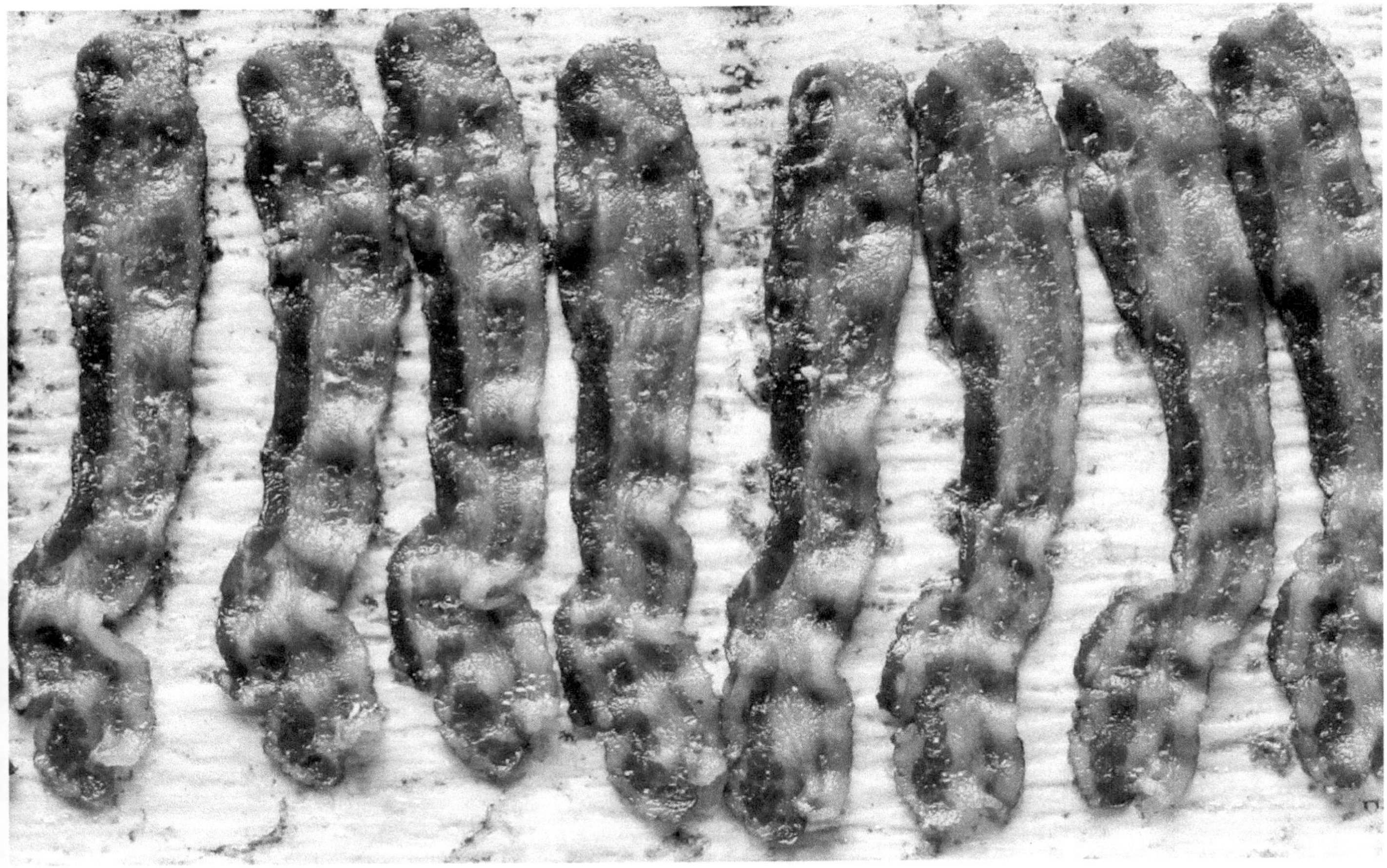

54 Roasted Leeks With Eggs

(Ready in about 40 minutes | Serving 2 | Difficulty: Easy)

Per serving: Kcal 1219, Fat: 124.6g, Net Carbs: 27.8g, Protein: 11.8g

Ingredients

- 3 green onions
- 2 leeks
- 2 tbsp. melted ghee (clarified butter)
- ¼ tsp. ground black pepper
- ½ tsp. sea salt

Avocado Vinaigrette:

- ¾ cup of light olive oil
- ⅛ tsp. red pepper flakes
- 1 ripe avocado, flesh scooped from the skin, pitted
- 1 lemon, juiced
- Ground black pepper and salt according to taste
- ¼ cup of red wine vinegar
- 1 tsp. olive oil
- ¼ cup of sliced, toasted almonds
- 2 eggs

Instructions

- Preheat oven to 400 degrees Fahrenheit.
- Green tops and bottom half-inch of the leeks should be discarded. Leeks can be sliced in half lengthwise.
- On a sheet tray, arrange the green onions and leeks. Drizzle ghee on top. Season with salt and pepper.
- For fifteen to twenty minutes in a preheated oven, roast till brown.
- In a food processor, thoroughly 3/4 cup olive oil, mix avocado, vinegar, lemon juice, pepper, and salt to make the vinaigrette

- In a skillet on medium-low flame, heat 1 tsp. oil for two to three minutes, or before whites are just set and the yolks are already runny, break eggs onto the opposite sides of the skillet.
- Remove the leeks and onions from the oven and put them on top with the sunny-side-up eggs. On top, sprinkle red pepper flakes and almonds. Finish with an avocado vinaigrette drizzle.

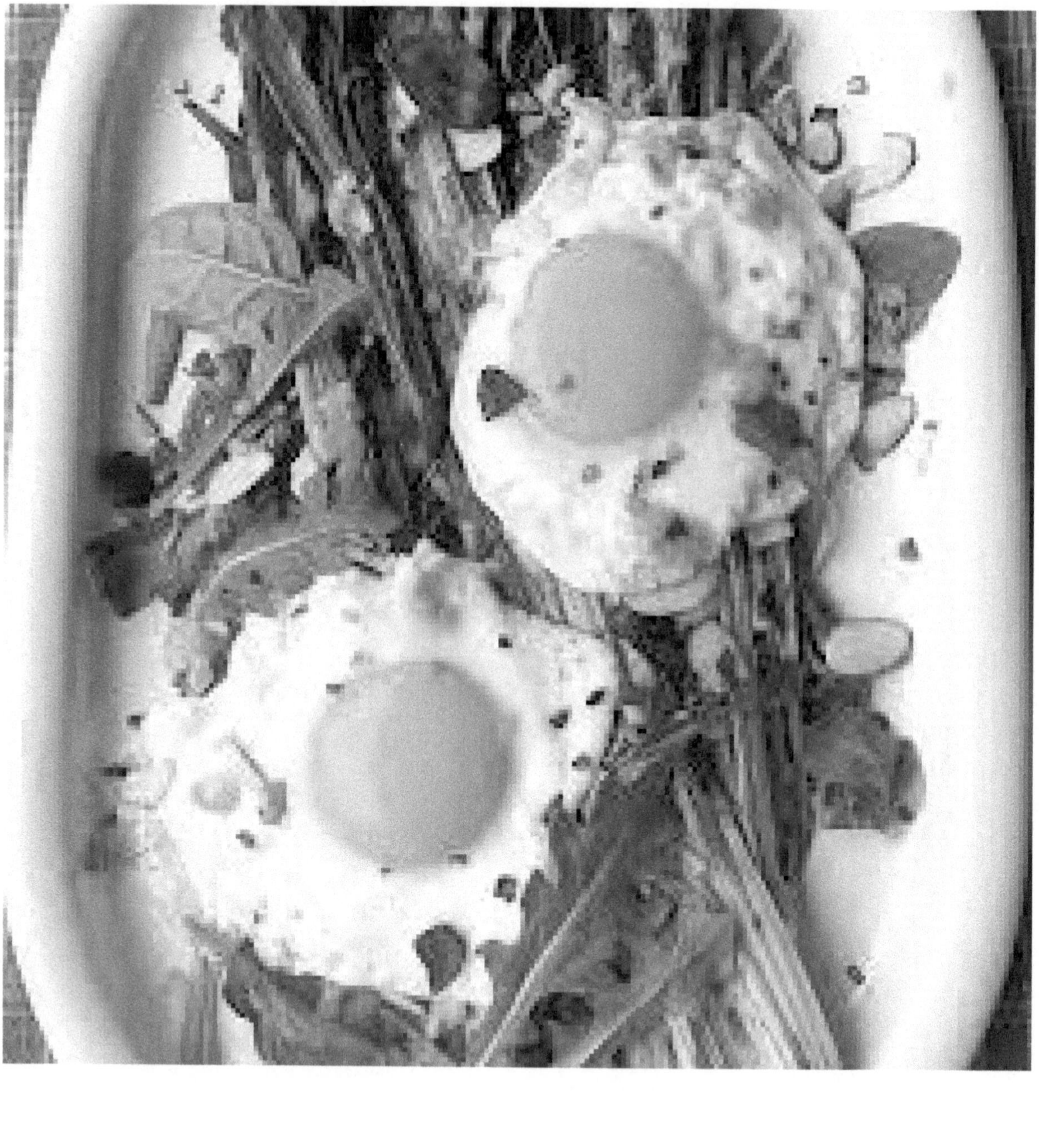

55 Gluten-Free Bagels

(Ready in about 30 minutes | Serving 6 | Difficulty: Easy)

Per serving: Kcal 364, Fat: 27.9g, Net Carbs: 9.7g, Protein: 20.9g

Ingredients

- 1 tbsp. baking powder, gluten-free
- 1 ½ cups of almond flour
- 2 eggs
- 1 tsp. garlic salt
- 2 oz. cream cheese, cubed
- 2 ½ cups of shredded mozzarella cheese

Instructions

- Preheat oven to 400 degrees Fahrenheit. Using parchment paper, line the baking sheet.
- In a mixing bowl, add the baking powder, garlic salt, and almond flour.
- In the microwave-safe bowl, mix mozzarella and cream cheese. Microwave for one minute, then remove and mix. Microwave for another minute, then take it off and stir until all is well combined. Working fast, stir the eggs and flour mixture into melted cheese mixture. Knead the dough by hand until it becomes a sticky dough. Continue kneading and pressing the dough for approximately two minutes or until it is fully uniform.
- The dough can be divided into six equal bits. Roll each one into the long log, then push the ends together to form a bagel shape and put it on the baking sheet that has been prepared.
- For ten to fourteen minutes in the preheated oven, bake till the bagels are golden.

55 Keto Zucchini Hash

(Ready in about 30 minutes | Serving 4 | Difficulty: Easy)

Per serving: Kcal 200, Fat: 17.9g, Net Carbs: 5g, Protein: g

Ingredients

- 3 tbsp. coconut oil
- 4 small zucchini, squeezed dry and grated
- 1 tbsp. butter
- 1 tsp. chili powder, or according to taste
- ⅓ cup of grated Parmesan cheese
- 1 tsp. sea salt
- 2 eggs, beaten
- 1 tsp. cayenne pepper (Optional)

Directions

- In a small skillet over medium flame, combine the coconut oil, butter, and zucchini. Add the chili powder, Parmesan cheese, cayenne pepper, and salt to a mixing bowl. Stir until the cheese has melted.
- Reduce the heat to a minimum and whisk in the eggs before thoroughly combined. Adjust to medium heat and fry, stirring and tossing sometimes, for almost fifteen minutes, or till the edges of hash are lightly browned.

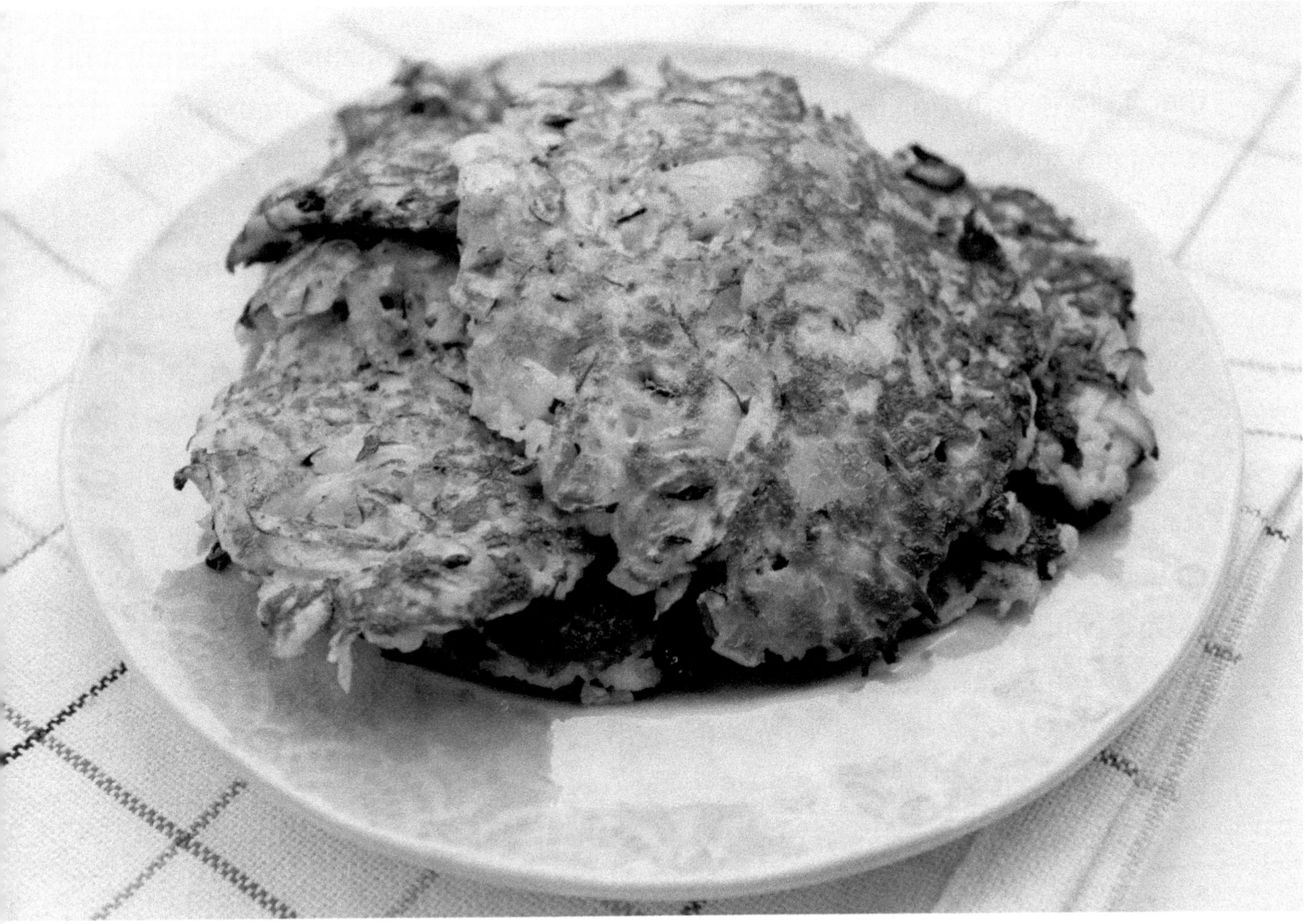

Conclusion

A keto diet may be a healthier option for certain people, although the amount of fat, carbohydrates, and protein prescribed varies from person to person. If you have diabetes, talk to the doctor before starting the diet because it would almost certainly need prescription changes and stronger blood sugar regulation. Are you taking drugs for high blood pressure? Before starting a keto diet again, talk to the doctor. If you're breastfeeding, you shouldn't follow a ketogenic diet. Be mindful that limiting carbs will render you irritable, hungry, and sleepy, among other things. However, this may be a one-time occurrence. Keep in mind that you can eat a balanced diet in order to obtain all of the vitamins and minerals you need. A sufficient amount of fiber is also needed. When the body begins to derive energy from accumulated fat rather than glucose, it is said to be in ketosis. Several trials have shown the powerful weight-loss benefits of a low-carb, or keto, diet. This diet, on the other hand, can be difficult to stick to and can exacerbate health issues in individuals who have certain disorders, such as diabetes type 1. The keto diet is suitable for the majority of citizens. Nonetheless, all major dietary modifications should be discussed with a dietitian or doctor. This is essentially the case with people who have inherent conditions. The keto diet may be an effective therapy for people with drug-resistant epilepsy. Though the diet may be beneficial to people of any age, teenagers, people over 50, and babies can profit the most because they can easily stick to it. Modified keto diets, such as the revised Atkins diet or the low-glycemic index diet, are safer for adolescents and adults. A health care worker should keep a careful eye on someone who is taking a keto diet as a treatment. A doctor and dietitian will maintain track of a person's progress, administer drugs, and test for side effects. The body absorbs fat and protein differently than it does carbohydrates. Carbohydrates have a high insulin reaction. The protein sensitivity to insulin is mild, and the quick insulin response is negligible. Insulin is a fat-producing and fat-conserving enzyme. If you wish to lose weight, consume as many eggs, chickens, fish, and birds as you want, satiate yourself with the fat, and then eat every vegetable that grows on the ground. Butter and coconut oil can be used instead of processed synthetic seed oils. You may be either a sugar or a fat burner, but not both.

Lightning Source UK Ltd.
Milton Keynes UK
UKHW051015240621
386081UK00009B/340

9 781803 061344